SIROLIMUS-ELUTING STENTS
FROM RESEARCH TO CLINICAL PRACTICE

Other Taylor & Francis Titles by
Patrick W Serruys

Handbook of Coronary Stents (1997, 1998, 2000, 2002)
Frontiers in Interventional Cardiology (1997)
Handbook of Vascular Brachytherapy (1998, 2000)
Coronary Stenting: Current Perspectives, *a Companion to the Handbook of Coronary Stents* (1999)
Coronary Lesions: A Pragmatic Approach (2001)
High Risk Cardiac Revascularization (2002)
Handbook of the Vulnerable Plaque (2004)
Handbook of Cardiac Cell Transplantation (2004)
Handbook of Drug Eluting Stents (2005)

SIROLIMUS ELUTING STENTS

FROM RESEARCH TO CLINICAL PRACTICE

Edited by

Patrick W Serruys MD PhD FACC FESC
Professor and Head
Department of Interventional Cardiology
Thoraxcenter
Erasmus University
Rotterdam
The Netherlands

and

Pedro A Lemos MD PhD
Interventional Cardiologist
Interventional Cardiology Service
Heart Institute (InCor)
University of São Paulo Medical School
São Paulo
Brazil

Foreword by
Martin B Leon MD
Chairman, Cardiovascular Research Foundation
Columbia University School of Medicine
New York NY
USA

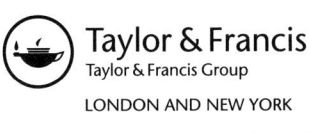

Taylor & Francis
Taylor & Francis Group

LONDON AND NEW YORK

A MARTIN DUNITZ BOOK

© 2005 Taylor & Francis, an imprint of the Taylor & Francis Group

First published in the United Kingdom in 2004
by Taylor & Francis, an imprint of the Taylor & Francis Group,
2 Park Square, Milton Park, Abingdon, Oxon, OX14 4RN

Tel.:   +44 (0) 1235 828600
Fax.:   +44 (0) 1235 829000
E-mail: info@dunitz.co.uk
Website: http://www.dunitz.co.uk

A CIP record for this book is available from the British Library.

Library of Congress Cataloging-in-Publication Data

Data available on application

ISBN 1 84184 492 6

Distributed in North and South America by
Taylor & Francis
2000 NW Corporate Blvd
Boca Raton, FL 33431, USA

Within Continental USA
Tel.: 800 272 7737; Fax.: 800 374 3401
Outside Continental USA
Tel.: 561 994 0555; Fax.: 561 361 6018
E-mail: orders@crcpress.com

Distributed in the rest of the world by
Thomson Publishing Services
Cheriton House
North Way
Andover, Hampshire SP10 5BE, UK
Tel.: +44 (0)1264 332424
E-mail: salesorder.tandf@thomsonpublishingservices.co.uk

Composition by Scribe Design, Ashford, Kent, UK
Printed by TJ International, Padstow, UK

To all the international fellows who have worked in the Thoraxcenter in the past (1976–2004) and I thank them for having made me wiser....

PWS

To my wife, Francine

PAL

CONTENTS

Contributors   ix

Foreword   xii

I   Sirolimus-Eluting Stents in the Clinical Practice: Concepts, and General Overview

1   Sirolimus-Eluting Stents as an Anti-Restenosis Device: Basic Concepts and Summary of Pivotal Studies   3
    Patrick W Serruys, Pedro A Lemos

2   Sirolimus-Eluting Stents in The 'Real World': The RESEARCH Registry Rationale and Study Design   15
    Pedro A Lemos, Patrick W Serruys, Ron T van Domburg

3   Unrestricted Utilization of Sirolimus-Eluting Stents for De Novo Coronary Lesions   23
    Pedro A Lemos, Patrick W Serruys, Ron T van Domburg

II Sirolimus-Eluting Stents for Patients at High Clinical Risk

4   Early Safety of Sirolimus-Eluting Stents for Patients with Acute Coronary Syndromes   35
    Pedro A Lemos, Chi-hang Lee, Patrick W Serruys

5   Sirolimus-Eluting Stents for Patients with Acute Myocardial Infarction   41
    Francesco Saia, Pedro A Lemos, Patrick W Serruys

6   Sirolimus-Eluting Stents for Patients with Impaired Renal Function   49
    Pedro A Lemos, Ron T van Domburg, Patrick W Serruys

7   Sirolimus-eluting Stents for Patients with Prior Coronary Bypass Graft Surgery   53
    Angela Hoye, Patrick W Serruys

8   Sirolimus-Eluting Stents for Left Main Coronary Artery Disease   59
    Chourmouzios A Arampatzis, Patrick W Serruys

9   Sirolimus-Eluting Stents for Patients with Multivessel Coronary Disease   67
    Chourmouzios A Arampatzis, Pedro A Lemos

10 Sirolimus-Eluting Stents for Elderlies   73
    Maniyal Vijayakumar, Pedro A Lemos, Patrick W Serruys

III Sirolimus-Eluting Stents for Patients at Special Anatomic Groups

11 Sirolimus-Eluting Stents for Chronic Total
    Occlusions   79
    Angela Hoye, Kengo Tanabe, Patrick W Serruys

12 Sirolimus-Eluting Stents for Very Small Coronary
    Vessels   87
    Pedro A Lemos, Patrick W Serruys

13 Sirolimus-Eluting Stents for Very Long Lesions   93
    Muzaffer Degertekin, Chourmouzios A Arampatzis,
    Pedro A Lemos

14 Sirolimus-Eluting Stents for Bifurcation Lesions   99
    Kengo Tanabe, Angela Hoye, Patrick W Serruys

15 Sirolimus-Eluting Stents for Coronary Narrowings
    <50% in Diameter   107
    Angela Hoye, Pedro A Lemos, Patrick W Serruys

16 Sirolimus-Eluting Stents for In-Stent Restenosis   113
    Francesco Saia, Patrick W Serruys

17 Post-Dilatation of Undersized Sirolimus-Eluting
    Stents   125
    Francesco Saia, Pedro A Lemos

IV Complications after Sirolimus-Eluting Stents

18 Thrombotic Stent Occlusion After Sirolimus-Eluting
    Stent Implantation   135
    Evelyn Regar, Pedro A Lemos, Patrick W Serruys

19 Morphology and Mechanisms of Restenosis After
    Sirolimus-Eluting Stents   141
    Pedro A Lemos, Francesco Saia

20 Predictors of Restenosis after Sirolimus-Eluting
    Stent Implantation in Complex Patients   147
    Pedro A Lemos, Dick Goedhart, Patrick W Serruys

21 Late Luminal Loss Response Pattern after Sirolimus-
    Eluting Stent Implantation or Conventional Stenting 153
    Pedro A Lemos, Ron T Van Domburg, Patrick W Serruys

22 Treatment of Post-Sirolimus-Eluting Stent Restenosis 157
    Pedro A Lemos, Carlos AG van Mieghem, Patrick W Serruys

vii

V   Costs of Sirolimus-Eluting Stents

23   Cost-Effectiveness of Sirolimus-Eluting Stents   165
Patrick W Serruys, Ben van Hout, Pedro A Lemos

References   169

Index   189

CONTRIBUTORS

Jiro Aoki MD
Research fellow
Catheterization Laboratory
Erasmus University Rotterdam
Erasmus Medical Center
Thoraxcenter
Rotterdam, The Netherlands

Chourmouzios A Arampatzis MD, PhD
Interventional Cardiologist
Euromedica Clinic
Thessaloniki, Greece

Marcel JBM van den Brand MD, PhD
Interventional Cardiologist
Catheterization Laboratory
Erasmus University Rotterdam
Erasmus Medical Center
Thoraxcenter
Rotterdam, The Netherlands

Paul Cummins RN
Research coordinator
Catheterization Laboratory
Erasmus University Rotterdam
Erasmus Medical Center
Thoraxcenter
Rotterdam, The Netherlands

Joost Daemen
Medical student
Erasmus University Rotterdam
Erasmus Medical Center
Rotterdam, Netherlands

Muzaffer Degertekin MD, PhD
Associate Professor of Cardiology
Department of Interventional Cardiology
Kosuyolu Heart & Research Hospital
Istanbul, Turkey

Ron T van Domburg PhD
Clinical Epidemiologist
Clinical Epidemiology Group
Erasmus University Rotterdam
Erasmus Medical Center
Thoraxcenter
Rotterdam, The Netherlands

Marco van Duuren
Medical student
Erasmus University Rotterdam
Erasmus Medical Center
Rotterdam, Netherlands

Gerrit-Anne van Es PhD
Director of Research & Development
Cardialysis B.V.
Rotterdam, The Netherlands

Pim de J Feyter MD, PhD
Professor, Non-Invasive Diagnosis of
Ischemic Heart Diseases
Interventional Cardiologist
Erasmus University Rotterdam
Erasmus Medical Center
Thoraxcenter
Rotterdam, The Netherlands

Willem J van der Giessen MD, PhD
Interventional Cardiologist
Catheterization Laboratory
Erasmus University Rotterdam
Erasmus Medical Center
Thoraxcenter
Rotterdam, The Netherlands

Dick Goedhart
Statistician
Cardialysis B.V.
Rotterdam, The Netherlands

Sjoerd H Hofma MD
Interventional Cardiologist
Catheterization Laboratory
Erasmus University Rotterdam
Erasmus Medical Center
Thoraxcenter
Rotterdam, The Netherlands

Ben A van Hout PhD
Professor of Medical Economics
Universitair Medisch Centrum
Julius Centrum
Utrecht, The Netherlands

Angela Hoye MB ChB, MRCP
Clinical Fellow
Catheterization Laboratory
Erasmus University Rotterdam
Erasmus Medical Center
Thoraxcenter
Rotterdam, The Netherlands

Richard E Kuntz MD, MSc
Cardiologist
Associate Professor of Medicine
Harvard Medical School
Brigham and Women's Hospital
Boston, Massachusetts, USA

Lee Chi-hang MBBS, MRCP
Associate Consultant Cardiologist
Cardiac Department
National University Hospital
Singapore

Pedro A Lemos MD, PhD
Interventional Cardiologist
Interventional Cardiology Service
Heart Institute (InCor)
University of São Paulo Medical School
São Paulo, Brazil

Jurgen MR Ligthart BSc
Senior technician
Catheterization Laboratory
Erasmus University Rotterdam
Erasmus Medical Center
Thoraxcenter
Rotterdam, The Netherlands

Wietze K. Lindeboom MSc
Statistician
Cardialysis B.V.
Rotterdam, The Netherlands

Tommy KK Liu
Medical student
Erasmus University Rotterdam
Erasmus Medical Center
Rotterdam, Netherlands

Eugene McFadden MB ChB, FRCPI
Interventional Cardiologist
Catheterization Laboratory
Erasmus University Rotterdam
Erasmus Medical Center
Thoraxcenter
Rotterdam, The Netherlands

Nestor Mercado MD, PhD
Medical resident
William Beaumont Hospital
Royal Oak, Michigan, USA

Carlos AG van Mieghem MD
Clinical fellow
Catheterization Laboratory
Erasmus University Rotterdam
Erasmus Medical Center
Thoraxcenter
Rotterdam, The Netherlands

Marie-Claude Morice MD
Interventional Cardiologist
Head of the Institut Cardiovasculaire
Paris Sud
Paris, France

William W O'Neill MD
Cardiologist
Corporate Chief of Cardiology
Director, Division of Cardiovascular
Disease
William Beaumont Hospital
Royal Oak, Michigan, USA

Andrew TL Ong MBBS FRACP
Research fellow
Catheterization Laboratory
Erasmus University Rotterdam
Erasmus Medical Center
Thoraxcenter
Rotterdam, The Netherlands

Evelyn Regar MD, PhD
Interventional Cardiologist
Catheterization Laboratory
Erasmus University Rotterdam
Erasmus Medical Center
Thoraxcenter
Rotterdam, The Netherlands

Arno Ruiter RN
Research coordinator
Catheterization Laboratory
Erasmus University Rotterdam
Erasmus Medical Center
Thoraxcenter
Rotterdam, The Netherlands

Francesco Saia MD, PhD
Interventional Cardiologist
Catheterization Laboratory
Institute of Cardiology
University of Bologna
Policlinico S. Orsola Malpighi
Bologna, Italy

Patrick W Serruys MD, PhD
Professor of Interventional Cardiology
Head of the Interventional Cardiology
Department
Erasmus University Rotterdam
Erasmus Medical Center
Thoraxcenter
Rotterdam, The Netherlands

Georgios Sianos MD, PhD
Interventional Cardiologist
Catheterization Laboratory
Erasmus University Rotterdam
Erasmus Medical Center
Thoraxcenter
Rotterdam, The Netherlands

Pieter C Smits MD, PhD
Interventional Cardiologist
Head of Interventional Cardiology
Department
Medical Center Rijnmond Zuid (MCRZ)
Rotterdam, The Netherlands

J Eduardo Sousa MD, PhD
Interventional Cardiologist
Head of Institute Dante Pazzanese of
Cardiology
São Paulo, Brazil

Kengo Tanabe MD
Cardiologist
Division of Cardiology
Mitsui Memorial Hospital
Tokyo, Japan

Maniyal Vijayakumar
Cardiologist
Amrita Institute of Medical Sciences &
Research Center
Cochin
India

FOREWORD

A remarkable undertaking

The introduction of drug-eluting stents represents a transformational and disruptive event in the three-stage evolutionary pathway of interventional vascular therapy. The first stage was the introduction and validation of balloon angioplasty as a percutaneous lesser-invasive treatment modality for patients with obstructive coronary disease. After a decade of iterative improvements in equipment design and operator technique, balloon angioplasty was still plagued by frequent dissections, disturbing early abrupt closure syndrome, inconsistent results in complex lesion subsets, and unacceptable clinical and angiographic mid-term recurrence. The second stage was the acceptance of coronary stents. Stents, serving as an endovascular scaffold, addressed many of the aforementioned problems and supplanted balloon angioplasty as the dominant default interventional therapy. However, stent implantation was associated with a significant wound healing response resulting in substantial intimal hyperplasia or tissue ingrowth. In-stent restenosis, often diffuse in nature and difficult to treat, rendered angioplasty unworthy as a definitive competitor compared to surgical revascularization in patients with complex coronary disease. Thus, restenosis, the Achilles heel of angioplasty since its inception, once again raised its ugly head and placed interventionalists in a subservient position in the overall scheme of coronary artery disease treatment dynamics.

Drug-eluting stents, by conquering restenosis, brings us to the third and final stage of our interventional odyssey. This elegant biotechnology solution to restenosis couples the stent backbone with potent site-specific pharmacotherapies delivered via biocompatible drug carrier vehicles. The near elimination of restenosis was indicated by early clinical trials, such as RAVEL, SIRIUS, TAXUS II and TAXUS IV. However, these landmark blinded, randomized clinical trials only exposed the 'tip of the iceberg'. It is estimated that these important proof-of-concept and regulatory approval studies for CYPHER™ and TAXUS™, by restricting entry criteria to simple and medium complexity lesions and patients, only constituted approximately 15% of the patients eligible for treatment with drug-eluting stents in the 'real world'.

Clearly, what was needed immediately after the commercial approval of the first drug-eluting stent, was a comprehensive analysis of safety and efficacy during the unrestricted use of this new technology in a consecutive series of PCI patients. The subject of this book by Serruys, Lemos, and colleagues is the formal catalogue of the Rapamycin-Eluting Stent Evaluated at Rotterdam Cardiology Hospital (RESEARCH) registry. Although the concept of RESEARCH seems obvious in retrospect, few will appreciate the exhaustive efforts required to thoughtfully formulate and execute a consecutive case series (compared with recent historical controls at the same institution) in 'all comers' with complex coronary disease. This study was not treated as a typical single center registry, but more like a formal randomized clinical trial. Prospective statistical models were developed, pre-specified endpoints were defined, clinical follow-up was obtained in everyone (with angiographic follow-up in high risk lesion subsets), and clinical event committees were assigned to adjudicate safety and efficacy endpoints. RESEARCH was 'a remarkable undertaking' and the global interventional community should be indebted to the authors and colleagues for the flawless implementation, analysis, and publication of the RESEARCH dataset.

Exactly what is RESEARCH and what have we learned? In perspective, RESEARCH has become both an overall assessment of a prospective group of patients compared with retrospective controls *and* a series of embedded substudies on important lesion and patient subsets. A large consecutive series of patients treated with sirolimus-eluting stents were compared with patients recently treated with conventional bare metal stent strategies. Importantly, we learned that in this 'real world' cohort of more complex lesions, the overall safety of sirolimus-eluting stents was reaffirmed and the clinical efficacy was similar to previously conducted randomized clinical trials. From the various 'high risk' substudies, we learned that safety and efficacy claims of sirolimus-eluting stents could be extended to acute MI lesions, small vessels, long lesions, chronic total occlusions, left main coronary lesions, multivessel disease, in-stent restenosis lesions, and bifurcation lesions.

Perhaps as important as the benefits demonstrated by drug-eluting stents in RESEARCH is the meticulous attention directed by Serruys, Lemos, and colleagues to limitations and shortcomings of these devices. Drug-eluting stents did not reduce overall mortality or myocardial infarctions (compared with bare metal stent controls) and the high one-year mortality observed in patients with chronic renal insufficiency was not attenuated in the sirolimus-eluting stent group. In diabetic patients, the benefit of sirolimus-eluting stents was present but diminished and diabetes was a predictor of subsequent in-segment restenosis. The benefit of sirolimus-eluting stents was also diminished in patients with ostial lesions (especially in bifurcation lesions) and in patients with in-stent restenosis (although comparable to vascular brachytherapy). Discontinuity of stent struts was determined as an important etiology of 'failure' (i.e. recurrence) after sirolimus-eluting stents and the treatment of in-stent restenosis within sirolimus-eluting stents was disappointing.

Interestingly, by emphasizing many of the shortcomings of drug-eluting stents, RESEARCH has helped to pave the future course of interventional device development leading to the next generation of drug-eluting stent concepts. Perhaps, different drugs, more potent drugs, or combinations of drugs will be required to finally 'cure' restenosis in the most difficult lesion subsets. Perhaps, new stent designs which ensure improved scaffolding and homogeneous drug distribution will be required to master bifurcation lesions. Perhaps, in the future, we will see more biocompatible and absorbable drug-eluting stent platforms. And perhaps, drug-eluting stents can also service the target end-organ by addressing other clinical imperatives, such as reperfusion injury after myocardial infarction. Finally, by arriving at a 'cure for restenosis', we humbly recognize the limitations of interventional vascular therapy. We haven't reduced mortality from cardiovascular disease and we haven't prevented myocardial infarctions, both crucial next goals as we redirect the efforts of experimental and clinical scientists.

RESEARCH was 'a remarkable undertaking' and the totality of studies and publications arising from this registry represents one of the most important contributions to our understanding of drug-eluting stents at the present time. Lemos and his colleagues, mentored by the mercurial Patrick Serruys, should be congratulated for these academic accomplishments. This book will undoubtedly become 'required reading' for serious students of drug-eluting stents and should serve as a model of superlative and timely evidence-based medicine answers to compelling clinical questions.

Martin B. Leon MD
Chairman, Cardiovascular Research Foundation
Columbia University School of Medicine
New York City

I SIROLIMUS-ELUTING STENTS IN THE CLINICAL PRACTICE: CONCEPTS, AND GENERAL OVERVIEW

1. SIROLIMUS-ELUTING STENTS AS AN ANTI-RESTENOSIS DEVICE: BASIC CONCEPTS AND SUMMARY OF PIVOTAL STUDIES

Patrick W Serruys, Pedro A Lemos

Introduction

In-stent restenosis has long been recognized as the main limitation of coronary stenting, with rates of restenosis as high as 50% being reported for some complex subgroups. Although a number of 'predictors' have been described and are helpful in characterizing 'high-risk' populations, the occurrence of restenosis remains largely unpredictable for a particular patient.[1–3] Moreover, in-stent restenosis in its more complex forms may recur in up to 80% of patients following percutaneous re-treatment with conventional techniques.[4] Although intracoronary brachytherapy has been proven effective in reducing the recurrence rate of in-stent restenosis, treatment failure still frequently occurs.

A large body of evidence has been accumulated in an attempt to understand the processes involved in restenosis. Differently from restenosis after balloon angioplasty, in which vessel shrinkage ('negative remodeling') contributes to the late luminal re-narrowing process, in-stent restenosis has been shown to be almost entirely due to neointimal tissue growth (Figure 1.1). The initial injury caused by the mechanical dilatation and stent implantation triggers a 'normal' healing vascular response that ultimately leads to neointimal formation, which, when excessive, may re-narrow the vessel lumen (restenosis). An array of local reparative processes have been shown to occur after the initial vascular trauma, involving platelets, inflammatory cells, smooth muscle cells, endothelial cells, and the secretion of a number of growth factors and cytokines.[5, 6]

Even though a large body of scientific knowledge is currently available on the mechanisms involved in the process of restenosis, numerous clinical trials utilizing systemic pharmacological agents failed to inhibit neointimal proliferation and to reduce in-stent restenosis. Similarly, several mechanical strategies addressed to optimize post-procedure luminal dimensions, a well-known predictor of late restenosis, also failed to significantly reduce the problem of restenosis.[7]

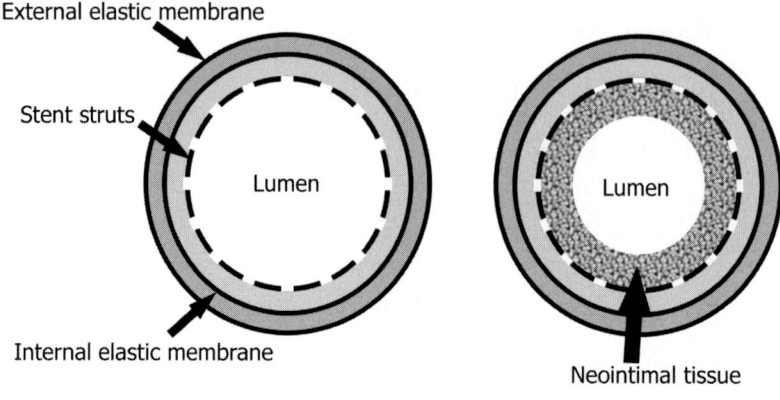

Figure 1.1 *The figure illustrates the process of restenosis after bare stent implantation, which is almost entirely due to proliferation of neointimal tissue towards the vessel lumen.*

More recently, however, drug-eluting stents have emerged as an effective therapeutic option to reduce the incidence of in-stent restenosis. The sirolimus-eluting stent was the first of such devices with proven capacity to decrease neointimal growth and ultimately reduce late restenosis. The present chapter will focus on describing the device structure, pre-clinical background, and the clinical information currently available from early studies and randomized trials conducted to date with the sirolimus-eluting stent.

Rationale for drug-eluting stents

A proposed explanation for the repeated failure of clinical pharmacological studies with systemically administered drugs is that these agents cannot reach sufficient tissue levels at the site of dilatation without increasing the risk of systemic side effects. In this regard, local administration offers advantages by applying the drug to the precise site of injury, therefore yielding very high concentrations of the active agent with low or negligible systemic levels.

Utilizing the stent itself as the platform for local drug delivery is an appealing approach. Coronary stents have been extensively proven to be safe and effective in mechanically alleviating coronary obstructions, with predictable

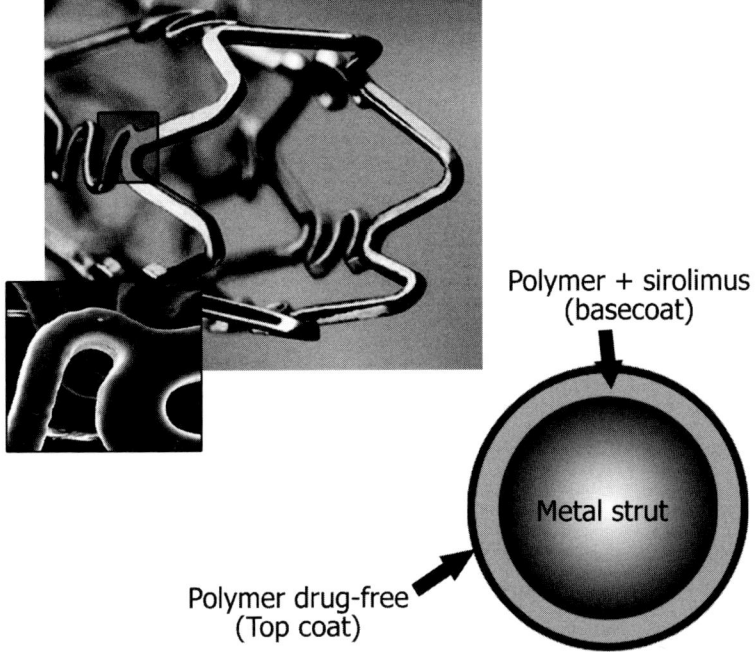

Figure 1.2 *The sirolimus-eluting stent. The platform utilized is the stainless steel Bx Velocity stent, which is covered by a 5–10 μm uniform blend of polymer + drug (basecoat). A topcoat of drug-free polymer is added to act as a diffusion barrier and control the release of drug.*

and stable short-term results in a wide range of clinical situations. By combining an agent with antiproliferative properties to a 'conventional' metallic stent, one is able to preserve the mechanical scaffolding properties of stenting while the active agent is administered to the very spot of vascular injury, with no time delay, with high local doses, and with the potential to control the kinetics (short- vs. long-course) and site (mural vs. luminal) of drug release, among other characteristics.

Sirolimus-eluting stent platform and carrier vehicle

The sirolimus-eluting stent (CYPHER™ stent [Cordis Corporation, a Johnson & Johnson company]) comprises an assembly of three main components: the metal stent platform, the drug carrier vehicle, and the pharmacologic agent sirolimus (Figure 1.2). The stent platform utilized is a third generation metal stent (Bx VELOCITY™ stent [Cordis Corporation, a Johnson & Johnson company]), which has been in clinical use for years before the introduction of the sirolimus-eluting stent. It is a stainless steel stent, with a strut thickness of 140 µm, and a closed-cell design. The stent is premounted in a delivery system and 5 nominal stent diameters are available: 2.25 mm to 3.0 mm (in 0.25-mm increments; 6-cell geometry) and 3.5 mm (7-cell geometry). The stent is available in lengths from 8 mm to 33 mm (with 5 mm increments).

The drug carrier vehicle utilized in the sirolimus-eluting stent is a mixed rate blend of the biologically stable polymers poly(ethylene-co-vinylacetate) (PEVA) and poly(butyl methacrylate) (PBMA). The stent is coated with a uniform 5–10 µm layer of the polymers, which has been shown in animal studies to be non-erodable and mechanically resistant. The sirolimus is mixed with the polymers and is released by the simple diffusion principle as soon as the stent is deployed and contact with the adjacent tissues and the blood is established.

The kinetics of the drug release from drug-eluting stents occurs as a function of several parameters, including the ratio of drug-polymer weights of the blend, the thickness of the polymeric coating, the molecular weight and water solubility of the drug, and the total drug dose load. Owing to the lipophilic nature of sirolimus, most of the drug is eluted to the adjacent vessel wall and not to the bloodstream, which increases the local bioavailability of the agent and minimizes the risk of systemic drug effects. In the sirolimus-eluting stent, a basecoat layer of the polymer-drug complex is added to the surface of the stent. In addition, a thin drug-free 'topcoat' of polymers is also assembled, which permits a more delayed release of the active agent. The sirolimus-eluting stent is designed to elute approximately 50% of the drug in the first week, 80% by the end of the first month, and 100% at 3 months from the stent deployment (Figure 1.3). In the early First-In-Man (FIM) registry, a subgroup of 15 patients received a fast-release formulation (<15-day drug release), which was not utilized in further trials nor is available for routine use.[8]

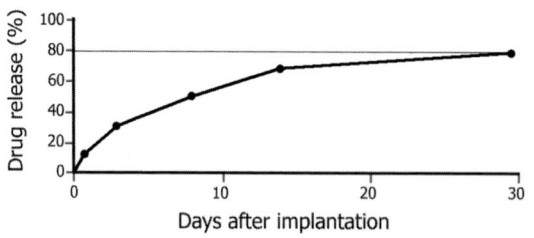

Figure 1.3 Drug release kinetics of sirolimus-eluting stents.

Sirolimus-eluting stents are loaded with a fixed amount of sirolimus per unit of metal surface area of 140 μg sirolimus/cm^2 ($\pm10\%$). The total sirolimus content of an 18-mm stent is 153 μg ($\pm10\%$) for the 6-cell stents and 180 μg ($\pm10\%$) for 7-cell stents.

Sirolimus

The local agent to be loaded to a stent with the aim of reducing neointimal proliferation should be one with cytostatic action that inhibits the complex cascade of events related to the 'healing' process that occurs after stent implantation.

Sirolimus (Rapamycin; Rapamune® Wyeth Laboratories) is a naturally occurring macrocyclic lactone with a potent immunosuppressive action, which was discovered in the 1970s and approved by the US Food and Drug Administration for use in renal transplant recipients in September 1999. Sirolimus is a highly lipophilic, low-molecular weight agent that inhibits cellular proliferation by blocking cell cycle progression at the G1 to S transition (Figure 1.4). Its action is mediated by binding to an intracellular receptor, the FK506 binding protein (FKBP12), which has been shown to be upregulated after vascular injury, such as stent implantation. The complex sirolimus-FKBP12 then binds a key regulatory kinase denominated mammalian Target Of Rapamycin (mTOR). The sirolimus-FKBP12-mTOR complex has

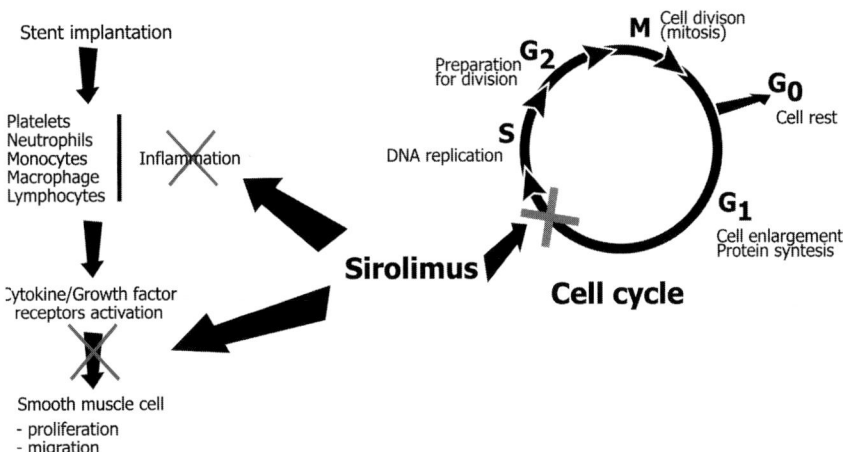

Figure 1.4 *Mechanism of action of sirolimus after stent implantation*

several important effects, including the inhibition of translation of a family of mRNAs that code for proteins essential for cell cycle progression.

The antiproliferative action of sirolimus has been shown to be associated to its capacity of preventing mitogen-induced downregulation of the cyclin-dependent kinase inhibitor p27Kip1.[9,10] In an alternative way, however, sirolimus may also lead to neointimal inhibition through a pathway that is independent of p27Kip1, a mechanism that was recently suggested by the demonstration that sirolimus reduces smooth muscle cell proliferation in p27Kip1(−/−) knockout mice.[9] As a result of these complex actions, sirolimus holds the cell cycle in late G1 phase (G1/S transition). In addition to its antiproliferative actions on smooth muscle cells, sirolimus has been shown to inhibit cytokine-driven (IL-2, IL-4, IL-7 and IL-15) T-cell proliferation and to interfere with macrophage function, actions that confer an anti-inflammatory effect to sirolimus (Figure 1.4).

Sirolimus-eluting stents have been shown to effectively inhibit neointimal proliferation in porcine and canine models in pre-clinical studies. At 1 week after the implantation, sirolimus-eluting stents reduced by 60% and 50% proliferating cell nuclear antigen and retinoblastoma protein expression respectively. At 4 weeks, the mean neointimal area of sirolimus-eluting stents was 50% smaller than the bare stent controls.[11]

Early clinical studies and summary of randomized trials with sirolimus-eluting stents

Sirolimus-eluting stents were first implanted in patients with coronary disease in the pioneer First-In-Man experience, which included 45 patients with relatively non-complex *de novo* lesions treated between December 1999 and February 2000.[8,12–16] Patients were treated in São Paulo, Brazil (n=30), and Rotterdam, The Netherlands (n=15) and received sirolimus-eluting stents in 2 formulations. Both formulations contained 140 μg of sirolimus per cm^2, but with different delivery kinetics (fast-release formulation [<15-day drug release], or slow release formulation [>28-day drug release]). Angiographic *in-stent* restenosis was not detected in any case up to 2 years and only one case had a 52% diameter stenosis proximal to the stent.[12,16] Two-year intravascular ultrasound examination showed only minimal neointimal proliferation, with 6.3±5.5% percent intimal hyperplasia within the stent in the fast release group (São Paulo), 7.5±7.3% in the slow-release group (São Paulo), and 4.4±3.1% in the slow-release group Rotterdam.[12,16] Moreover, the 2-year event-free survival was 90.1%, with no extra major events occurring between 2 and 3 years.[14]

Table 1.1. Randomized trials comparing bare metal stents with sirolimus-eluting stents – Study characteristics

	Study groups	Inclusion criteria	Exclusion criteria	Antiplatelet
RAVEL[17,18,136]	Polymer-coated sirolimus-eluting stent (n=120 pts) Bare stent (n=118 pts)	de novo lesion native vessel single lesion lesion length <18 mm vessel diameter 3–3.5 mm	total occlusion ostial thrombus containing lesion unprotected LMC with >50% stenosis evolving myocardial infarction left ventricular ejection fraction <30%	Aspirin lifelong Clopidogrel for 2 months
SIRIUS[19]	Polymer-coated sirolimus-eluting stent (n=533 pts) Bare stent (n=525 pts)	de novo lesion native vessel single lesion lesion length 15–30 mm vessel diameter 2.5–3.5 mm	total occlusion ostial thrombus con-taining lesion unprotected LMC with >50% stenosis myocardial infarction <48 hours left ventricular ejection fraction <25% bifurcation multivessel stenting	Aspirin lifelong Clopidogrel for 3 months
E-SIRIUS[20]	Polymer-coated sirolimus-eluting stent (n=175 pts) Bare stent (n=177)	de novo lesion native vessel single lesion lesion length 15–32 mm vessel diameter 2.5–3.0mm	total occlusion ostial thrombus con-taining lesion unprotected LMC with >50% stenosis evolving myocardial left ventricular ejection fraction <25% infarction bifurcation multivessel stenting	Aspirin lifelong Clopidogrel for 2 months
C-SIRIUS[21]	Polymer-coated sirolimus-eluting stent (n=50 pts) Bare stent (n=50 pts)	de novo coronary lesion single lesion Stable or unstable angina or docu-mented silent ischemia Lesion length 15–32 mm Vessel diameter 2.5–3.0 mm	total occlusion Recent MI (<24 hours) Unprotected LM disease Ostial location Angiographic evidence of thrombus Pretreatment with devices other than balloon LV ejection fraction <25%	Aspirin lifelong Clopidogrel for 2 months
pts=patients				

Table 1.2. Randomized trials comparing bare metal stents with sirolimus-eluting stents – Patient and procedural characteristics

	Diabetics (%)	AMI admission (%)	Multivessel disease (%)	LAD (%)	LM (%)	IIbIIIa (%)	ACC/AHA Lesion type C (%)	Chronic total occlusion (%)	Stents/pt (%)	Bifurcation stenting (%)
RAVEL[17,18,136]										
Sirolimus	16	0	NA	49	0	10.1	0	0	1.0±0.3	0
Bare stent	21	0	NA	51	0	9.5	0	0	1.1±0.3	0
SIRIUS[19]										
Sirolimus	25	0	42	44	0	60	26	0	1.4±0.7	0
Bare stent	28	0	41	43	0	59	21	0	1.4±0.6	0
E-SIRIUS[20]										
Sirolimus	19	0	NA	57	0	14	NA	0	*	0
Bare stent	27	0	NA	56	0	18	NA	0	*	0
C-SIRIUS[21]										
Sirolimus	24	0	46	36	0	58	30	0	1.38±0.57†	0
Bare stent	24	0	34	40	0	48	16	0	1.66±0.94	0

AMI=acute myocardial infarction; LAD=left anterior descending artery; LM=left main coronary
* overlapping stents in 34% (sirolimus) vs. 31% (bare stent)
† $p < 0.05$ vs. control

Table 1.3. Randomized trials comparing bare metal stents with sirolimus-eluting stents – Quantitative Angiography Analysis

| | Pre-procedure | | Post-procedure | | Follow-up | | | | |
	RD (mm±SD)	length (mm±SD)	DS (%±SD)	MLD (mm±SD)	time (months)	DS (%±SD)	MLD (mm±SD)	Restenosis (%)	Late loss (mm±SD)
RAVEL[17,18,136]*									
Sirolimus	2.60±0.54	9.56±3.33	11.9±5.9‡	2.43±0.41	6	14.7±7.0 ‡	2.42±0.49 ‡	0 ‡	-0.01±0.33 ‡
Bare stent	2.64±0.52	9.61±3.18	14.0±6.8	2.41±0.40	6	36.7±18.1	1.64±0.59	26.6	0.80±0.53
SIRIUS[19]†									
Sirolimus	2.79±0.45	14.4±0.58	16.1±9.7	2.38±0.45	8	23.6±16.4 ‡	2.15±0.61 ‡	8.9 ‡	0.24±0.47 ‡
Bare stent	2.81±0.49	14.4±0.58	16.2±8.5	2.4±0.46	8	43.2±22.4	1.60±0.72	36.3	0.81±0.67
E-SIRIUS[20]†									
Sirolimus	2.60±0.37‡	14.9±5.4	18.2±9.6	2.17±0.39	8	24.7±14.7 ‡	1.97±0.48 ‡	5.9 ‡	0.19±0.39 ‡
Bare stent	2.51±0.37	15.1±6.5	18.0±9.1	2.10±0.39	8	48.3±23.4	1.29±0.61	42.3	0.80±0.57
C-SIRIUS[21]†									
Sirolimus	2.65±0.30	14.5±6.3	17.5±7.1	2.23±0.35	8	20.5±10.3	2.15±0.35‡	2.3‡	0.12±0.35‡
Bare stent	2.62±0.35	12.6±5.2	18.5±10.0	2.17±0.37	8	47.8±24.5	1.39±0.69	52.3	0.79±0.74

*In-stent quantitative coronary angiography
†In-segment quantitative coronary angiography (includes the 5-mm proximal and distal edges)
‡ p<0.05 vs. control

Table 1.4. Randomized trials comparing bare metal stents with sirolimus-eluting stents – Clinical Outcomes

Study	Follow-up (months)	Death (%)	Myocardial infarction (%)	Target lesion revascularization (%)	Any event (%)	Stent thrombosis (%)*
RAVEL[17,18,136]	12					
Sirolimus		1.7	3.3	0*	5.8*	0
Bare stent		1.7	4.2	22.9	28.8	0
SIRIUS[19,22]	12					
Sirolimus		1.3	3.0	4.9*‡	8.3*	0.4
Bare stent		0.8	3.4	20.0	22.3	0.8
E-SIRIUS[20]	9					
Sirolimus		1.1	4.6	4.0*‡	8.0*	1.1
Bare stent		0.6	2.3	20.9	22.6	0
C-SIRIUS[21]	9					
Sirolimus		0	2	4.0*‡	4.0*	2.0
Bare stent		0	4	18.0	18.0	2.0

*rates of angiographically documented stent thrombosis
† p≤0.05 vs. control
‡ 'clinically-driven' re-intervention

Four randomized trials comparing the outcomes of patients treated with sirolimus-stents and conventional bare stents have been concluded to date, and are summarized in Tables 1.1, 1.2, 1.3, and 1.4.[17–21] The Randomized Study with the Sirolimus-Eluting Bx Velocity Balloon-Expandable Stent in the Treatment of Patients with de Novo Native Coronary Artery Lesions (RAVEL) trial included 238 patients with single non-complex de novo lesions. At six months' follow-up, the angiographic restenosis rate of the treated group was zero and the loss in minimal lumen diameter was zero. The clinical outcomes were significantly better among patients treated with sirolimus stents, with 94% of patients being free of any major cardiac events at 1 year (compared to 71% in the bare stent group; p<0.01).[18] Recently, data from the RAVEL trial with a more prolonged follow-up period have shown maintenance of the initial results, with a 2-year event-free survival of 90%.[17]

The subsequent SIRolImUS-Eluting Bx Velocity™ Balloon-Expandable Stent (SIRIUS) trial, which randomized 1101 patients with *de novo* lesions to sirolimus or bare stents, confirmed the clinical efficacy of sirolimus-eluting stents.[19,22] In-stent binary restenosis (within the margins of the stent) was reduced by 91% (3.2% vs. 35.4%; p<0.01) and in-segment restenosis (including the stented portion and the 5 mm segments proximal and distal to the stent) was reduced by 75% (8.9% vs. 36.3%; p<0.01).[19] At 12 months, the incidence of major adverse events was significantly lower in the sirolimus group (8.3% vs. 22.3%; p<0.01), mainly due to a decrease in the need of target lesion revascularization (4.9% vs. 20.0%; p<0.01). Prolonged follow-up data (up to 2 years) were recently presented and showed sustained benefit of sirolimus-eluting stent implantation in the SIRIUS trial.[23] The recently published E-SIRIUS trial has enrolled 352 patients with longer lesions and smaller vessels than the RAVEL and SIRIUS trials.[20] Nevertheless, the 8-month in-stent restenosis rate was 3.9% in the sirolimus and 41.7% in the bare stent group (p<0.01). Similarly, the incidence of in-segment restenosis (5-mm edges included) was significantly reduced (5.9% vs. 42.3%; p<0.01). The 9-month incidence of major cardiac events was 8% vs. 22.6% in the sirolimus and bare groups (p<0.01). In the C-SIRIUS trial, which randomized 100 patients to sirolimus or conventional stenting, in-stent restenosis was not detected in any patient after sirolimus-eluting stent implantation.[21] In this trial, in-segment restenosis was 2.3% (versus 52.3% for controls; p<0.01). Differently from the previous trials, in the C-SIRIUS trial direct stenting was allowed (at the discretion of the operator), which did not affect the incidence of restenosis.

2. SIROLIMUS-ELUTING STENTS IN THE 'REAL WORLD': THE RESEARCH REGISTRY RATIONALE AND STUDY DESIGN

Pedro A Lemos, Patrick W Serruys,
Ron T. van Domburg

Introduction

Recently, sirolimus-eluting stents (SES) have been shown to markedly reduce the incidence of angiographic restenosis.[8,12–16,18–22] In these devices, the metallic stent platform surface is loaded with biologically inert and mechanically resistant polymers blended with the antiproliferative agent sirolimus, which is progressively eluted from the assembly after implantation in a controlled manner. This way, percutaneous treatment can be carried out without loss of acute efficacy (since the mechanical properties of the endovascular prosthesis are maintained), while the stent itself acts as an anti-neointimal growth device.

In the first clinical experience with SES, the First-In-Man (FIM) study,[8,12–16] no cases of restenosis were detected in a series of 45 patients, with persistent neointimal inhibition demonstrated up to 4 years (J.E. Sousa, MD, PhD. Personal communication. ACC meeting 2004). These findings have been further confirmed in randomized trials comparing SES with conventional bare stents.[18–22] In the RAndomized study with the sirolimus-eluting Bx VElocity balloon-expandable stent in the treatment of patients with de novo native coronary artery Lesions (RAVEL),[18] there were no cases of binary angiographic restenosis in patients treated with SES implantation. In the SIRolImUS-eluting Bx velocity balloon expandable stent (SIRIUS),[19,22] in the E-SIRIUS,[20] and in the C-SIRIUS[21] trials, (in-segment) restenosis occurred in 2.3% to 8.9% of cases in the SES groups, which was significantly lower than the restenosis rates seen among patients treated with conventional stents (p<0.001 for all studies).

After the first results of the FIM experience,[8,12–16] the early results of the RAVEL trial,[18] and the more recent SIRIUSs trials,[19–22] SES have progressively received clinical approval by official regulatory agencies. Since the first half of 2002, these devices have been available for routine use in Europe, Asia, and

South America, and since 2003 in the U.S. However, from the above-mentioned trials, relatively scarce information could be derived on the clinical performance of SES for many patient subsets frequently seen in the so-called 'real world'. The effects of SES implantation in unselected patients with more complex clinical and anatomic presentations, such as those commonly treated in the daily practice, remained largely unexplored.

The Rapamycin-Eluting Stent Evaluated At Rotterdam Cardiology Hospital registry (RESEARCH) was designed to investigate the impact of sirolimus-eluting stent implantation utilized as the default strategy on the outcomes of patients treated in the 'real world' of interventional cardiology. The basic concept of the RESEARCH registry consisted of comparing the outcomes of patients treated before and after the introduction of sirolimus-eluting stents. To accomplish this objective, sirolimus-eluting stents were instituted as the device of choice for all patients, with no specific clinical or anatomical restrictions. Furthermore, sirolimus-eluting stents were introduced swiftly and replaced the metallic bare stents on April 16, 2002 (less than one week after SES became commercially available in Europe), thereby permitting the identification of two distinct and separate groups of patients primarily distinguished by the interventional strategy applied (bare stent or SES implantation).

Patient population

RESEARCH is a single-center registry that enrolled all consecutive patients treated with percutaneous intervention, who were separated into two distinct cohorts: patients treated before and after the utilization of SES (Cypher; Johnson & Johnson-Cordis unit, Cordis Europa NV, Roden, The Netherlands) as the default strategy for every percutaneous procedure (Figure 2.1).

Patients enrolled in the first 6 months after the introduction of SES (from April 2002 to October 2002) and the corresponding group of patients treated in the 6 months immediately prior (from April 2002 to October 2001) comprised the main patient population analyzed in most reports derived from this experience. Nevertheless, unrestricted SES utilization continued beyond October 2002 and some substudies from RESEARCH utilized extended enrolment periods (greater than 6 months) in order to augment the sample size of patients treated with SES. On average, approximately 130 patients were treated with percutaneous intervention each month during RESEARCH.

Figure 2.1 illustrates the study design and the patient population included in both phases of RESEARCH. In the first 6 months after SES introduction, a total of 798 consecutive patients underwent percutaneous interventions, with

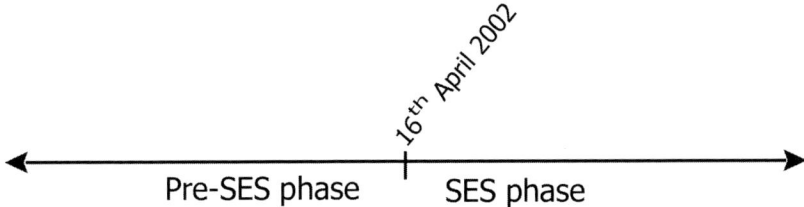

SES phase (6-month enrollment)

798 consecutive patients treated with percutaneous interventions
- 631 patients treated with at least one sirolimus-eluting stent (SES)
- 563 patients treated exclusively with SES
- 68 patients treated with bare stents and SES in the same procedure *

Pre-SES phase (6-month enrollment)

806 consecutive patients treated with percutaneous interventions
- 718 patients treated with bare stents.

* Non-utilization of SES was due to unavailability of an appropriate SES size (diameter or length) in 77% of cases

Figure 2.1 *Study design and 6-month enrolment patient of RESEARCH.*

631 patients (79.1%) being treated with at least one sirolimus-eluting stent. From these, 563 patients (89.2%) were treated exclusively with SES and 68 patients (10.8%) were treated with bare stents and SES in the same procedure. Non-utilization of SES was due to unavailability of an appropriate SES size (diameter or length) in 77% of cases (at the initiation of the RESEARCH registry, SES were available in diameters from 2.25 mm to 3.00 mm and lengths of 8 mm, 18 mm, and 33 mm) or inclusion in other studies in 5%. During the 6-month period that preceded the SES introduction (pre-SES control phase), a total of 806 consecutive patients underwent percutaneous interventions. From these, 718 patients (89.1%) were treated with bare stents.

Table 2.1 shows the main exclusion criteria for the four randomized trials conducted to date with SES. Also, the proportion of patients enrolled in RESEARCH who had the corresponding exclusion criterion is depicted. It is noteworthy that the vast majority (68%) of patients studied in RESEARCH would not be included in the previous randomized trials on the basis of their more complex profile.

Table 2.1. Main exclusion criteria for the RAVEL, SIRIUS, E-SIRIUS, and C-SIRIUS trials and the respective proportion of patients included in the RESEARCH (treatment only with SES)

Exclusion criteria for RAVEL, SIRIUS, E-SIRIUS, and C-SIRIUS	Proportion of patients in the RESEARCH treated only with SES
Multivessel stenting	28%
Very long lesion stenting (stented length > 36 mm)	19%
Acute myocardial infarction	18%
Very small vessels (stent ≤ 2.25 mm)	15%
Bifurcation stenting (stent + stent)	16%
Chronic total occlusion	8%
Renal impairment (creat >1.5 mg/dl)	6%
Age > 80 years	5%
Main stem stenting	3%
Saphenous vein graft stenting	3%
Any of the above	68%

Procedures and post-intervention medications

All interventions were performed according to current standard guidelines[24] and the final interventional strategy was left entirely to the discretion of the operator. Angiographic success was defined as residual stenosis <30% by visual analysis in the presence of TIMI 3 grade flow. Periprocedural glycoprotein IIb/IIIa inhibitors and antithrombotic medications were used according to the operator's decision. All patients were advised to maintain lifelong aspirin. One-month clopidogrel treatment (75 mg/d) was recommended for patients treated in the pre-SES phase. For patients treated with SES, clopidogrel was prescribed for 3 months, unless one of the following was present (in which case clopidogrel was maintained for at least 6 months): multiple SES implantation (>3 stents), total stented length >36 mm, chronic total occlusion, bifurcations, and in-stent restenosis treatment.

Endpoint definitions and clinical follow-up

The primary outcome was the occurrence of major adverse cardiac events, defined as

18

(1) Death,
(2) Non-fatal myocardial infarction, or
(3) Target vessel revascularization.

Myocardial infarction was diagnosed by a rise in the creatine kinase level to more than twice the upper normal limit with an increased creatine kinase-MB. Target lesion revascularization was defined as a repeat intervention (surgical or percutaneous) to treat a luminal stenosis within the stent or in the 5-mm distal or proximal segments adjacent to the stent. Target vessel revascularization was defined as a re-intervention driven by any lesion located in the same epicardial vessel. Thrombotic stent occlusion was angiographically documented as a complete occlusion (TIMI flow 0 or 1) or a flow limiting thrombus (TIMI flow 1 or 2) of a previously successfully treated artery.

Information about the in-hospital outcomes was obtained from an electronic clinical database for patients maintained in our institution and by review of the hospital records for those discharged to referring hospitals (patients were referred from a total of 14 local hospitals). Post-discharge survival status was obtained from the Municipal Civil Registries. All repeat interventions (surgical and percutaneous) and re-hospitalizations were prospectively collected during the follow-up. Questionnaires were sent at 6 months and 1 year to all living patients with information regarding post-discharge anginal status, medication usage, and the occurrence of clinical events. Furthermore, a psychological questionnaire was sent and included forms with the SF-36 quality of life,[25] the Hospital Anxiety and Depression Scale (HADS) anxiety and depression score[26] and the Type D personality score.[27] The referring physician and institutions, as well as the general practitioner, were directly approached whenever necessary for additional information. For patients who went abroad, an effort was made to contact the local civil registries of their new residencies. Patients lost to follow-up were considered at risk until the date of last contact, at which point they were censored.

During follow-up, coronary angiography was obtained as clinically indicated by symptoms or documentation of myocardial ischemia. Additionally, late angiographic evaluation was also obtained from pre-defined patient subsets (see below) in the SES group. No angiographic re-study was performed in the pre-SES group. Owing to the well-known effect of angiographic re-evaluation in increasing the incidence of repeat revascularization,[28] all re-interventions were retrospectively adjudicated and classified as clinically driven or non-clinically driven by a group of clinicians not involved in the treatment of the particular patient analyzed. Clinically driven repeat revascularization was defined as any intervention motivated by a significant luminal stenosis (>50% diameter stenosis) in the presence of anginal symptoms and/or proven myocardial ischemia in the target vessel territory by non-invasive testing.

Angiographic follow-up

Patients receiving sirolimus-eluting stents were considered as candidates for angiographic re-evaluation if presenting at least one of the following:

(1) Treatment of acute myocardial infarction
(2) Treatment of in-stent restenosis
(3) Utilization of very small sirolimus-eluting stent (2.25-mm nominal diameter)
(4) Treatment of the left main coronary artery
(5) Treatment of chronic total occlusion (of more than 3 months)
(6) Total adjacent stented segment longer than 36 mm, and
(7) Bifurcation stenting (sirolimus-eluting stent implanted in the both the main vessel and the side branch).

Patients with the aforementioned characteristics who had not undergone repeat intervention in the first month and not presented any formal medical contraindication for angiographic re-study were considered eligible for angiographic follow-up at 6 to 8 months. Coronary angiograms performed prematurely owing to clinical indications were used as the follow-up angiography if performed after 4 months or if restenosis were detected. In other cases, a second angiogram was obtained between 6 and 8 months. Importantly, although all patients were approached for angiographic follow-up, patient refusal was not considered as an exclusion criterion to be enrolled in the RESEARCH. Angiographic re-study was not requested for non-residents in The Netherlands. During the first 6 months of enrolment, a total of 362 consecutive patients had at least one high-risk criterion from the list above (57% of all patients treated with sirolimus-eluting stents in the period). From these, 2 patients moved to another country, 10 patients had died by 6-month follow-up, 6 patients had repeat intervention before 30 days (surgical or percutaneous), and 3 patients were considered to have a medical contra-indication to the angiographic follow-up (one patient with previous stroke and disabling dementia, one patient with severe allergic contrast reaction at the index procedure, and one patient with end-stage hepatic failure which was due to auto-immune hepatitis). From the remaining 341 patients, angiographic re-evaluation at 204±34 days was obtained from 238 patients (70% of eligible patients), who compose the population of the angiographic substudy of the RESEARCH.

Quantitative coronary angiography

Quantitative coronary angiographic analysis was performed as previously described, utilizing a validated computer-based edge-detection system (CASS

II, Pie Medical, Maastricht, The Netherlands).[29] Interpolated reference diameter, minimal luminal diameter, and diameter stenosis were obtained at baseline, post-stenting, and at follow-up. In-stent restenosis was defined by diameter stenosis >50% and was classified as in-stent if inside the stent, or in-segment if located within the stented segment plus the 5-mm segments distal or proximal to the stent margins (the latter were classified as *edge restenosis*).[19] Restenosis at an ostial location (within 3 mm of the vessel origin) was classified as *in-stent*, unless clearly located outside the limits of the SES. Acute gain was defined as the difference between minimal luminal diameter post- and pre-procedure. Late loss was calculated as the difference between the minimal luminal diameter immediately after the procedure and the minimal luminal diameter at six months. Loss index was defined as the ratio between late loss and acute gain.

In summary

RESEARCH is a single-center registry that evaluated the impact of sirolimus-eluting stents utilized as the device of choice in the daily practice. From April 2002, sirolimus-eluting stent implantation has been routinely used as the default strategy for all percutaneous interventions, from which outcomes were compared to patients treated with conventional techniques in the period immediately before. Among the consecutive series of cases that comprised the patient population enrolled in the RESEARCH registry, the vast majority (~70%) would not be included in earlier SES clinical trials on the grounds that they were considered to be 'high risk' patients. In this context, RESEARCH represented a unique source of information about the clinical performance of the sirolimus-eluting stents in patients treated in the so-called 'real world' of interventional cardiology.

3. UNRESTRICTED UTILIZATION OF SIROLIMUS-ELUTING STENTS FOR DE NOVO CORONARY LESIONS

Pedro A Lemos, Patrick W Serruys,
Ron T. van Domburg

Introduction

Sirolimus-eluting stents (SES) have been shown effective in the context of randomized trials with elective patients. However, the effects of SES implantation in more complex, unselected patients, such as those frequently found in daily practice, cannot be directly extrapolated from the findings of the available randomized trials. It is worth noting that the occurrence of restenosis in a small, but relevant proportion of patients in the SIRIUS trial, occurred mainly in patients with diabetes, small vessels, and long lesions,[30] characteristics frequently found in daily practice. This contrasts with the 'zero' restenosis rate of the RAVEL trial,[18] which included patients with lower risk profile. It is therefore reasonable to speculate whether the performance of sirolimus-eluting stents would be maintained in a clinical scenario where treatment of patients at high risk for restenosis is the rule rather than the exception.

In this chapter, the impact of sirolimus-eluting stents on the outcomes of patients treated in the 'real world' of interventional cardiology is analyzed. The safety and the effectiveness of a strategy of unrestrictive utilization of sirolimus-eluting stent is compared to a strategy utilizing conventional bare stent implantation.

Patient population

In the first 6 months enrolment in the RESEARCH registry, a total of 508 patients with *de novo* lesions were treated exclusively with SES and are analyzed in the present chapter (SES group). These patients were compared to a group of consecutive patients treated with bare stents for *de novo* lesions in the preceding 6 months (pre-SES group). In order to better match the vessel sizes treated in the 2 study groups, patients receiving bare metal stents larger than 3.5-mm were excluded from this analysis. This cutoff value, instead of 3.0-mm diameter stents, was chosen because of the post-dilatation policy applied in the SES group, which extended the utilization of SES to patients with 3.5-mm vessels by visual estimation. Also, patients treated with bare stents smaller than 2.25 mm (minimum stent diameter for SES) were not included. In total, 450 consecutive patients comprised the pre-SES group. For a detailed description of the RESEARCH design, the reader is referred to Chapter 2.

Baseline and procedural characteristics

Baseline and procedural characteristics of the two study groups are shown in Table 3.1 and Table 3.2. Overall, approximately half of the patients in both groups were admitted with acute coronary syndromes and diabetes was present

Table 3.1. Baseline characteristics of patients treated with conventional bare stents before the introduction of SES (Pre-SES group) and patients treated exclusively with SES implantation (SES Group). (From Lemos et al.[30a])

	Pre-SES Group (n=450)	SES Group (n=508)	P-value
Male, %	72	68	0.4
Age, years±SD	61±11	61±11	0.7
Diabetes, %	15	18	0.3
Non-insulin dependent	11	12	0.7
Insulin-dependent	4	6	0.2
Hypertension, %	48	41	0.2
Hypercholesterolemia, %	55	56	1.0
Current smoking, %	34	31	0.3
Previous MI, %	40	30	<0.01
Previous angioplasty, %	18	19	0.8
Previous bypass surgery, %	8	9	0.5
Single-vessel disease, %	52	46	0.05
Multivessel disease, %	48	54	0.05
Clinical presentation			0.7
Stable angina, %	48	45	
Unstable angina, %	35	37	
Acute myocardial infarction, %	18	18	
Cardiogenic shock, %*	12	10	0.7

*relative to patients with acute MI

Table 3.2. Angiographic and procedural characteristics of patients treated with conventional bare stents before the introduction of SES (Pre-SES group) and patients treated with SES implantation (SES Group). (From Lemos et al.[30a])

	Pre-SES Group (n=450)	SES Group (n=508)	P-value
Treated Vessel			
Left anterior descending, %	59	59	0.8
Left circumflex, %	33	32	0.7
Right coronary artery, %	34	39	0.2
Left main coronary, %	2	3	0.6
Bypass graft, %	2	3	0.2
Lesion type			
Type A, %	20	22	0.4
Type B1, %	32	31	0.7
Type B2, %	50	49	0.8
Type C, %	30	43	<0.01
Glycoprotein IIbIIIa inhibitor, %	33	19	<0.01
Clopidogrel prescription, months±SD	2.9±2.0	4.0±2.0	<0.01
Bifurcation stenting, %	8	16	<0.01
Number of stented segments ±SD	1.8±0.9	2.0±1.0	<0.01
Number of implanted stents ±SD	1.9±1.2	2.1±1.4	<0.01
Individual stent length ≥ 33 mm, %	10	35	<0.01
Total stented length per patient, mm±SD	30±20	39±28.7	<0.01
Nominal stent diameter ≤ 2.5 mm, %	23	36	<0.01
Post-dilatation with a balloon ≥ 0.5 mm larger, %	19	55	<0.01
Angiographic success of all lesions,%	97	97	1.0

in 16% of cases. Patients treated with SES had significantly more multivessel disease, more type C lesions, more bifurcation stenting, more segments stented, and more stents used. Also, in the SES group, long stents and stents with smaller diameters were more frequently deployed. Periprocedural administration of glycoprotein IIb/IIIa inhibitors was more frequent in the pre-SES phase (33% vs. 19%; p<0.01). The angiographic success rate was similar in both groups.

Clinical outcomes

Complete follow-up information was available for 99.1% of patients (mean follow-up period, 405 days). There were no significant differences between the SES group and the pre-SES group in the incidence of major adverse cardiac

Table 3.3. 30-day outcomes of patients treated with conventional bare stents before the introduction of SES (Pre-SES group) and patients treated exclusively with SES implantation (SES Group). (From Lemos et al.[30a])

	Pre-SES Group (n=450)	SES Group (n=508)	P-value*
Death, %	2.0	1.6	0.6
Non-fatal myocardial infarction, %	1.6	0.8	0.4
Target lesion revascularization, %	1.8	1.0	0.4
Target vessel revascularization, %†	2.2	1.0	0.2
Any event, %	4.2	3.0	0.3
Stent thrombosis, %‡	1.6	0.4	0.1

*by Fisher's exact test
†Includes target lesion revascularization
‡Angiographically documented stent thrombosis requiring repeat intervention

events during the first month (3.0% vs. 4.2% respectively; p=0.3) (Table 3.3). Target vessel revascularization at 30 days was 1.0% (n=5) in the SES group and 2.2% (n=10) in the pre-SES group (p=0.2), which included emergency bypass surgery in 2 patients (0.4%) in the SES group and in 2 cases (0.4%) in the pre-SES group (p=1.0) and early 'redo' target vessel revascularization (e.g. residual dissection or compromised side branch in patients with continuing symptoms) in 1 patient (0.2%) in the SES group and in 1 patient (0.2%) in the pre-SES group (p=1.0). In the remaining cases, 30-day repeat intervention was due to angiographically documented stent thrombosis in 2 patients (0.4%) in the SES group and in 7 patients (1.6%) in the pre-SES group (p=0.1). No further thrombotic stent occlusion was observed in the late follow-up.

At 1 year, the cumulative incidence of death was similar between both groups (3.4% for the SES group vs. 4.3% for the pre-SES group; hazard ratio (HR) 0.78 [95% CI 0.41–1.52]; p=0.5). Also, the incidence of death or myocardial infarction did not differ between the SES and the pre-SES groups (5.4% vs. 6.3% respectively; HR 0.84 [95% CI 0.50–1.40]; p=0.8). However, patients treated with SES had significantly less death, myocardial infarction or target vessel revascularization at 1 year (9.7% vs. 14.8% in the pre-SES group; HR 0.62 [95% CI 0.44–0.89]; p=0.008) (Figure 3.1), mainly due to a decrease in the need for target vessel revascularization in the SES group (5.1% vs. 10.9% in the pre-SES group; HR 0.49 (95% CI 0.29–0.82); p=0.007). Specifically, treatment with SES was associated with a marked reduction in clinically driven repeat interventions at 1 year (3.7% vs. 10.9% in the pre-SES group; HR 0.35 (95% CI 0.21–0.57); p<0.001) (Figure 3.2).

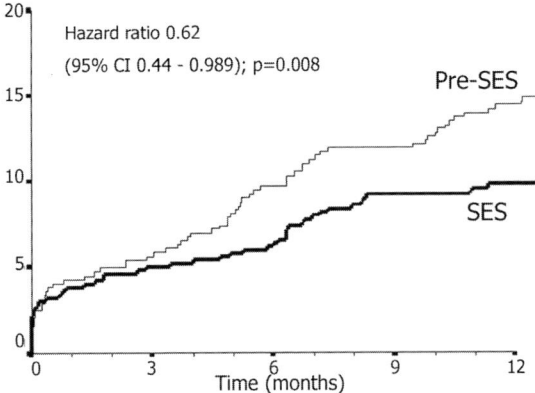

Figure 3.1 *One-year incidence of death, myocardial infarction or target vessel revascularization in patients treated with bare stents before the introduction of SES (Pre-SES group) and in patients treated exclusively with SES implantation (SES Group). (From Lemos et al.[30a])*

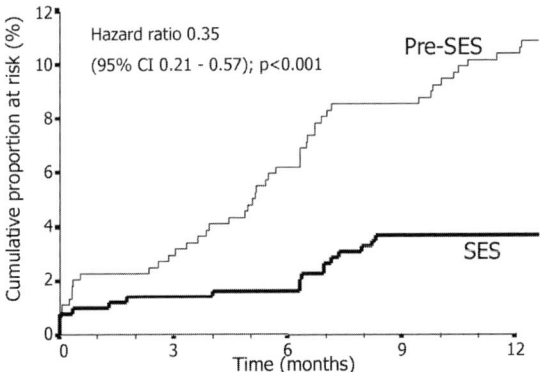

Figure 3.2 *One-year cumulative risk of clinically driven target vessel revascularization in patients treated with bare stents before the introduction of SES (Pre-SES group) and in patients treated exclusively with SES implantation (SES Group). (From Lemos et al.[30a])*

Predictors of adverse events

The impact of SES implantation on the risk of subsequent clinically driven target vessel revascularization in specific subsets is shown in Figure 3.3. Sirolimus-eluting stent implantation was associated with a risk reduction that ranged from 28% to 79% across the subgroups evaluated. However, the benefit

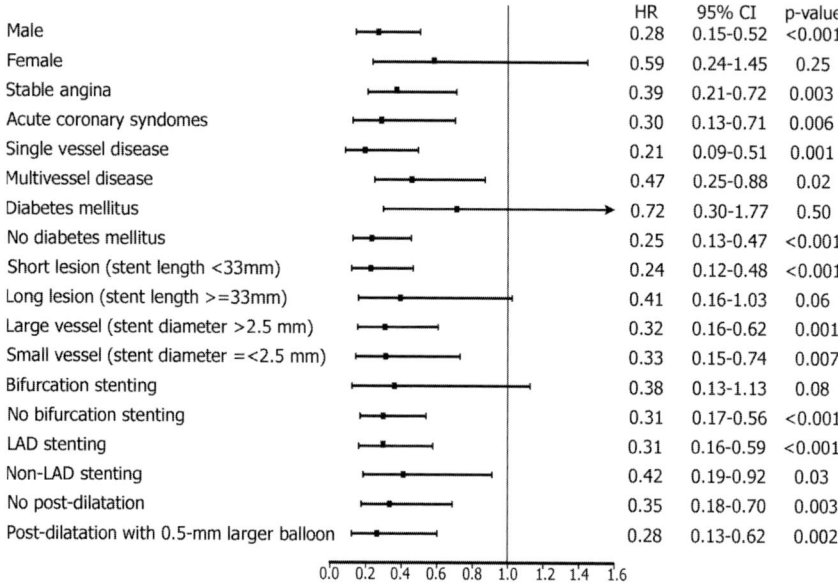

	HR	95% CI	p-value
Male	0.28	0.15-0.52	<0.001
Female	0.59	0.24-1.45	0.25
Stable angina	0.39	0.21-0.72	0.003
Acute coronary syndomes	0.30	0.13-0.71	0.006
Single vessel disease	0.21	0.09-0.51	0.001
Multivessel disease	0.47	0.25-0.88	0.02
Diabetes mellitus	0.72	0.30-1.77	0.50
No diabetes mellitus	0.25	0.13-0.47	<0.001
Short lesion (stent length <33mm)	0.24	0.12-0.48	<0.001
Long lesion (stent length >=33mm)	0.41	0.16-1.03	0.06
Large vessel (stent diameter >2.5 mm)	0.32	0.16-0.62	0.001
Small vessel (stent diameter =<2.5 mm)	0.33	0.15-0.74	0.007
Bifurcation stenting	0.38	0.13-1.13	0.08
No bifurcation stenting	0.31	0.17-0.56	<0.001
LAD stenting	0.31	0.16-0.59	<0.001
Non-LAD stenting	0.42	0.19-0.92	0.03
No post-dilatation	0.35	0.18-0.70	0.003
Post-dilatation with 0.5-mm larger balloon	0.28	0.13-0.62	0.002

Figure 3.3 *Hazard ratio of 1-year clinically driven target vessel revascularization in subgroups of patients according to baseline and procedural characteristics. (From Lemos et al.[30a])*

of SES did not reach statistical significance in women (HR 0.59 [95% CI: 0.24–1.45]; p=0.25) and diabetics (HR 0.72 [95% CI: 0.30–1.77]; p=0.50). Patients treated with bifurcation stenting (HR 0.38 [95% CI: 0.13–1.13]; p=0.08) and patients receiving 33-mm or longer stents (HR 0.41 [95% CI: 0.16–1.03]; p=0.06) presented a strong trend to have better outcomes with SES implantation. In the other subgroups, SES utilization significantly decreased the need of repeat intervention (Figure 3.3). Importantly, the post-dilatation strategy applied in the present study did not influence the clinical benefit of SES implantation. The magnitude of the risk reduction was similar between patients treated with post-dilatation (HR 0.28 [95% CI: 0.13–0.62]; p=0.002) or without post-dilatation (HR 0.35 [95% CI: 0.18–0.70]; p=0.003).

Multivariate Cox proportional hazards analysis identified sirolimus-eluting stent utilization to be independently associated with a reduced risk of adverse clinical events (Table 3.4). After adjustment for other independent variables, SES significantly decreased the risk of clinically driven target vessel revascularization (adjusted HR 0.33 [95% CI 0.20–0.56]; p<0.01) and the risk of major adverse cardiac events (adjusted HR 0.55 [95% CI 0.38–0.80]; p<0.01).

Table 3.4. Multivariate predictors of adverse events (Cox proportional hazards model).* (From Lemos et al.[30a])

	HR	95% CI	p-value
Major adverse cardiac events*			
SES utilization	0.55	0.38–0.80	<0.01
Cardiogenic shock	4.73	2.31–9.70	<0.01
Diabetes mellitus	1.62	1.09–2.43	0.02
Left main stenting	2.93	1.48–5.82	<0.01
Utilization of at least one 33-mm long stent	1.54	1.02–2.33	0.04
Clinically driven target vessel revascularization			
SES utilization	0.33	0.20–0.56	<0.01
Acute coronary syndromes†	0.51	0.32–0.80	<0.01
Number of stented segments	1.25	1.01–1.55	0.04
Diabetes mellitus	1.81	1.10–2.99	0.02

CI=confidence interval; HR=hazard ratio; SES=sirolimus-eluting stent
*Major adverse cardiac events: death, myocardial infarction, or target vessel revascularization
†Unstable angina or acute myocardial infarction at admission

Interpretation of the findings

Sirolimus-eluting stent implantation has been shown to markedly decrease the incidence of in-stent restenosis in the context of randomized trials.[18,30] However, these studies have enrolled relatively non-complex patient populations referred for elective intervention. As a consequence, the findings from these studies cannot be directly extrapolated to many patients treated in the everyday practice, where complex, non-elective cases are the rule, rather than the exception. In the present chapter it is shown that, sirolimus-eluting stents implantation is associated with a reduction in the rates of repeat revascularization and major adverse cardiac events at one-year in a consecutive, unselected cohort of patients. Sirolimus-eluting stent implantation resulted in a relative reduction of 51% in the overall rate of target vessel revascularization and of 65% in the rate of clinically driven target vessel revascularization.

The present series compared a strategy of unrestricted usage of sirolimus-eluting stents with conventional approaches utilizing bare stents in the pre-sirolimus-eluting stent 'era'. Although the two study groups were consecutively included over a total period of only one year, some important differences were noted in the interventional strategy applied. Patients in the sirolimus-eluting stent phase were treated with a less restrictive interventional approach, with a significant increase in the number and length of stents implanted, number of coronary segments dilated, bifurcation stenting, and decrease in the diameter of the stents. Possibly, this change in practice may reflect the early recognition by the operators that the acute results, even in this complex population, were maintained in medium-term. Also, it may reflect an attempt to accomplish more complete lesion coverage and ensure uniform drug-delivery over the entire diseased segment, since stent discontinuity and edge injury have been recognized to be associated with post-SES restenosis (see Chapter 18). Moreover, the higher complex profile of patients treated with SES (e.g. high rates of multivessel disease, type C lesions, bifurcations) may translate a change in the decision-making process promoted by the availability of sirolimus-eluting stents. Although both study groups differed in some baseline and procedural characteristics, which may somewhat limit an unbiased comparison between them, it is worth noting that most, if not all, differences would be traditionally expected to increase the incidence of late complications in the SES-treated patients. Nevertheless, the treatment effect of sirolimus-eluting stents was significantly higher than bare stents, remaining virtually unaffected after adjustment for procedural characteristics.

The reduction of adverse events after sirolimus-eluting stent implantation in the present series is lower than that observed in the RAVEL trial, where no binary angiographic restenosis was diagnosed.[18] The present findings more closely resembles those seen in the SIRIUS trial (75% reduction in clinically driven target lesion revascularization), in which patients with higher risk profiles were included.[30] Compared to the RAVEL study, the relative decline in effectiveness in the SIRIUS trial and in the RESEARCH study may have been related to the complexity of the procedures included. Although SES implantation markedly reduced the risk of subsequent revascularization in most subsets, the benefit of the new treatment did not reach statistical significance in some subgroups in our series. Indeed, the presence of diabetes and treatment of long lesions were shown to independently increase the incidence of complications. These findings highlight the need of further analyses with enlarged number of patients in order to fully estimate the clinical impact of SES in these patients. Also, whether the outcomes of higher risk subgroups can be improved with refinements in the procedural techniques remain to be established.

Importantly, the reduction of late complications was accomplished without any increase in unexpected sudden events. The present results show that sirolimus-eluting stent implantation in complex patients is safe, with no increase in acute device-related adverse events. The incidence (0.4%) and timing (within the first month) of documented thrombotic stent occlusion in the SES group was compatible with the current results with conventional bare metal stents. The utilization of IIb/IIIa inhibitors and clopidogrel differed between both study groups. However, these differences did not significantly influence the clinical outcome in our study. Nevertheless, it should be noted that these agents were not uniformly used across the various patient subsets, being mainly used in cases at a higher risk of complications, which may have blunted the overall positive effect of these drugs.

Although restenotic lesions have been shown to be amenable to treatment by sirolimus-eluting stents,[31,32] the treatment of *de novo* lesions may be considered as the main field of application of the new device. In this regard, RESEARCH was conducted to evaluate the use of sirolimus-eluting stent as a prophylactic strategy in preventing, rather than treating, in-stent restenosis in the 'real world'.

Some patients have not been treated with the sirolimus-eluting stents during the time period of the study. However, in most instances, this was due to unavailability of large-diameter sirolimus-eluting stents. As large vessels have been shown to present a lower risk of restenosis,[30] it is quite possible that the non-inclusion of patients with larger vessels may have resulted in an underestimation of the overall treatment effect in the present report.

In conclusion, these findings demonstrate that unrestricted utilization of sirolimus-eluting stents in the 'real world' is safe and effective in reducing the need of further revascularization and the incidence of major adverse cardiac events after one year, as compared to patients treated with bare stent implantation in the period immediately before.

II Sirolimus-Eluting Stents for Patients at High Clinical Risk

4. EARLY SAFETY OF SIROLIMUS-ELUTING STENTS FOR PATIENTS WITH ACUTE CORONARY SYNDROME

Pedro A Lemos, Chi-hang Lee, Patrick W Serruys

Introduction

Percutaneous intervention has been increasingly demonstrated to reduce the risk of adverse events in patients with acute coronary syndromes (ACS).[33,34] Several technical and medical advancements have all contributed to improve the results of angioplasty in this population. However, patients with acute coronary disease still present a higher risk for early events than chronic stable patients, possibly because of an increased propensity for thrombotic complications in the first days after the intervention.[35–37] Sirolimus has been described to decrease endothelial function *in vitro*[38] and to affect platelet physiology.[39–41] Moreover, impaired local vascular healing with delayed endothelialization and late fibrin persistence has also been raised as potential concerns.[42, 43] Therefore, the present chapter aims to describe the 30-day safety of patients admitted with unstable angina or acute myocardial infarction treated with sirolimus-eluting stents (SES).

Patient population

This chapter evaluates the 30-day outcomes of all 198 consecutive patients with unstable angina or acute myocardial infarction (MI) treated exclusively with SES during the first 4 months of the RESEARCH registry. A Control Group for comparison comprised 301 consecutive patients with ACS treated with bare stent implantation during the last 4 months prior to the initiation of the RESEARCH registry. Patients with unstable angina were categorized according to the Braunwald classification.[44] Procedures performed in the first 24 hours of an acute MI were classified as rescue or primary angioplasty, if

Table 4.1. Baseline and procedural characteristics of patients treated with bare stents versus patients treated with sirolimus-eluting stents. (Reprinted from Lemos et al.[44a] With permission from American College of Cardiology Foundation.)

	Bare Stent (n=301)	SES (n=198)	p-value
Age, years±SD	60±12	62±11	0.21
Male sex, %	75	68	0.10
Diabetes, %	12	18	0.07
Hypercholesterolemia	48	49	0.93
Current smoking, %	38	38	0.85
Hypertension, %	63	63	0.93
Previous MI, %	45	28	<0.01
Previous angioplasty, %	18	21	0.56
Previous CABG, %	10	9	0.64
Coronary artery disease, %			0.12
Single-vessel disease	44	51	
Multivessel disease	56	49	
Unstable angina, %	68	68	1.0
Braunwald classification, %*			
Class I to III-A	5	4	0.61
Class I and II-B	45	42	0.65
Class III-B	21	22	0.78
Class I and II-C	14	9	0.23
Class III-C	15	22	0.12
Acute MI, %	32	32	1.0
Cardiogenic shock †	13	13	1.0
Rescue angioplasty †	23	5	<0.01
Primary angioplasty †	77	95	<0.01
Peak CKMB, UI/L±SD ‡	317±256	217±236	0.04
IIBIIIA inhibitor, %	42	27	<0.01
Vessel treated, %			
LMC	3	4	0.60
LAD	58	59	0.85
LCx	31	29	0.69
RCA	39	36	0.64
Bypass	6	5	0.84
Lesion type A/B1, %	42	44	0.71
Lesion type B2/C, %	78	78	1.0
Number of treated segments (±SD)	1.8±0.9	1.8±0.9	1.00
Total stented length, mm±SD	28±13	29±15	0.30
Bifurcation stenting	5	13	<0.01
Angiographic success of all lesions, %	97	96	0.48

SES=sirolimus-eluting stent; MI=myocardial infarction; CABG=coronary artery bypass-graft surgery; LMC=left main coronary; LAD=left anterior descending artery; LCx=left circumflex artery; RCA=right coronary
*relative to the number of patients with unstable angina; total sum may not result 100% due to rounding
†relative to the number of patients with acute MI
‡Upper limit of normal = 24 UI/L

preceded or not by (failed) intravenous thrombolysis respectively. Patients treated after 24 hours but before discharge of an episode of myocardial infarction were classified as post-MI unstable angina (Braunwald Class C).

Baseline and procedural characteristics

Clinical and procedural characteristics of the 499 patients analyzed in this chapter are depicted in Table 4.1. As compared to controls, patients treated with SES had more frequently primary angioplasty (95% vs. 77%; p<0.01), more bifurcation stenting (13% vs. 5%; p<0.01), less previous MI (28% vs. 45%; p<0.01), and less glycoprotein IIb/IIIa inhibitor utilization (27% vs. 42%; p<0.01) (Table 4.1). Also, peak creatine kinase MB was lower for acute MI patients treated with SES (217±236 UI/L vs. 317±256 UI/L; p=0.04) (Table 4.1). Procedural angiographic success was achieved in all attempted lesions in a similar proportion of cases in the SES and the control groups (96% vs. 97% respectively, p=0.48) (Table 4.1).

30-day Outcome

The 30-day outcomes of the SES and control groups are shown in Table 4.2. There were no differences in the incidence of adverse events between patients treated with bare stents and those treated with SES (30-day MACE rate 6.1%

Table 4.2. Incidence of adverse events at 30 days in patients treated with bare stents versus patients treated with sirolimus-eluting stents. (Reprinted from Lemos et al.[44a] With permission from American College of Cardiology Foundation.)

	Bare Stent (n=301)	SES (n=198)	p-value
Death, %	3.0	3.0	1.0
Non-fatal MI, %	1.0	3.0	0.17
TLR, %	2.7	1.0	0.33
TVR (includes TLR), %	2.7	1.0	0.33
Total MACE %	6.6	6.1	0.85
Thrombotic stent occlusion, %	1.7	0.5	0.41

MACE=major adverse cardiac event; MI=myocardial infarction; SES=sirolimus-eluting stent; TLR=target lesion revascularization; TVR=target vessel revascularization

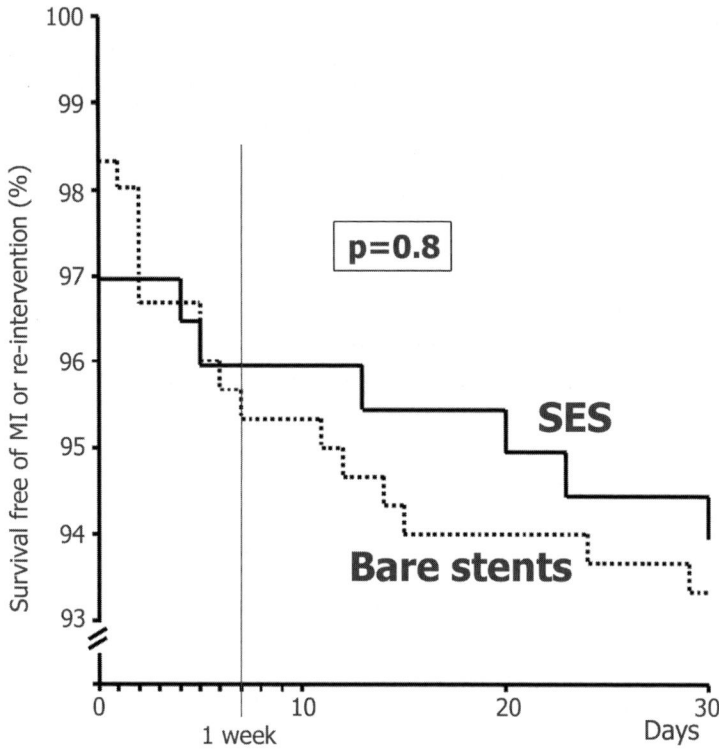

Figure 4.1 Survival free of myocardial infarction or re-intervention during the first month for patients treated with sirolimus-eluting stents or with bare stents. There is no difference in early complications between the groups. Note that most events occurred within the first week in both groups. (Reprinted from Lemos et al.[44a] With permission from American College of Cardiology Foundation.)

vs. 6.6%, respectively; p=0.8), with most complications occurring in the first week after the procedure (Figure 4.1). Stent thrombosis occurred in 1 patient (0.5%) in the SES group and in 5 patients (1.7%) in the control group (p=0.4) (Table 4.2). Four characteristics were identified as multivariate independent predictors of 30-day major adverse cardiac events (MACE): multivessel disease (odds ratio [OR] 4.4 [95% CI: 1.8–10.8]; p<0.01), cardiogenic shock (OR 3.9 [95% CI: 1.2–12.8]; p=0.02), acute MI at presentation (OR 3.3 [95% CI: 1.4–7.6]; p<0.01), and right coronary angioplasty (OR 0.4 [95% CI: 0.2–0.9]; p=0.04). Sirolimus-eluting stent utilization was not associated with an increased risk of complications (OR 1.0 [95% CI: 0.4–2.2]; p=0.97). Figure 4.2 illustrates a case of a patient with high-risk unstable angina treated with SES.

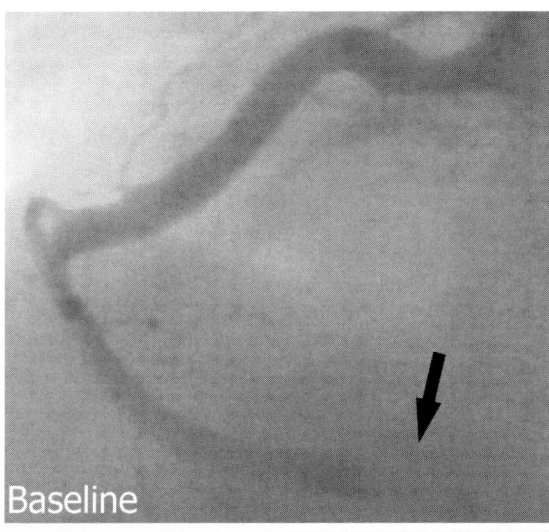

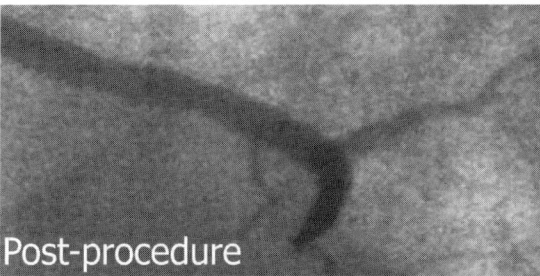

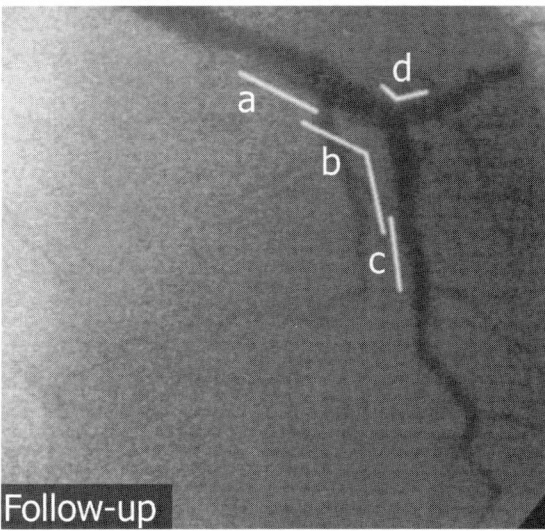

Figure 4.2 High-risk unstable angina treated with sirolimus-eluting stents. The figure shows the coronary angiogram of a patient admitted with post-infarction rest angina, with a totally occluded right coronary artery (top) and evidence of intraluminal thrombus (arrow). Four sirolimus-eluting stents were implanted at the distal bifurcation of the right coronary artery utilizing a 'crushing' technique (3.0 × 18 mm [a]; 2.5 × 33 mm [b]; 2.25 × 18 mm [c]; 2.25 × 8 mm [d]). The patient was pre-treated with abciximab and there were no post-procedure complications. At 6-month follow-up, there was no angiographic evidence of neointimal proliferation (bottom).

Interpretation of the findings

As compared to conventional bare stents, utilization of SES in unselected patients with acute MI or unstable angina was observed to be safe at 30 days, with similar rates of procedural success and early adverse events. Patients treated with SES differed in some aspects from that included in the control group. Control patients presented more rescue angioplasty for failed thrombolysis (instead of primary angioplasty), which could have increased the risk of events in this group. Conversely, SES patients were more frequently treated for bifurcation lesions, a well-known risk factor for periprocedural complications.[45,46] Moreover, glycoprotein IIb/IIIa inhibitors were less commonly used in patients treated with SES, which may have posed these patients to a higher procedural risk.[47] It seems unlikely that the lower utilization of glycoprotein IIb/IIIa blockers in these group could be explained by a lower risk profile perceived during the procedure, since both the control and SES populations were equally composed predominantly by patients with acute MI or high grade unstable angina, with no significant difference in their diabetic status. Nevertheless, after adjusting for baseline and procedural differences, the type of stent used, either bare stent or SES, was not significantly associated with the occurrence of early adverse events.

Recently, sirolimus has been reported to reduce endothelium-dependent relaxation in vitro in a porcine model, although the authors did not ruled out an effect of the drug vehicle.[38] Additionally, sirolimus has been described to increase platelet aggregation and secretion in transplant recipients.[41] However, recent studies have demonstrated that this drug efficiently blocks the synthesis of Bcl-3, a regulatory protein expressed when platelets adhere to collagen via integrin $\alpha_{IIb}\beta_{III}$.[39,40,48] Regardless of these contradictory laboratory findings, SES were not associated with clinically relevant device-related complications in our series, with no modification of the risk profile for procedural failure or event occurrence.

Patients treated with SES presented a similar timing of post-procedural complications as compared to controls, with most events occurring in the first days after the procedure, a typical pattern previously reported after bare stent implantation.[36,37] In this context, a relatively delayed hazardous effect of the drug leading to an increase in 'late' thrombotic complications after the first week was not observed in our patients.

In conclusion, sirolimus-eluting stent implantation for patients with acute coronary syndromes was safe, with early outcomes comparable to conventional bare metal stents. The maintenance of the excellent short-term results already achieved with conventional techniques is a key point for the validation of SES as a useful strategy in treatment of patients with acute coronary syndromes.

5. SIROLIMUS-ELUTING STENTS FOR PATIENTS WITH ACUTE MYOCARDIAL INFARCTION

Francesco Saia, Pedro A Lemos, Patrick W Serruys

Introduction

This chapter describes the impact of sirolimus-eluting stent (SES) implantation on the long-term outcomes of patients with acute myocardial infarction. The clinical and angiographic outcomes of this subset of patients have not been examined in any randomized trial to date and the experience derived from the RESEARCH might be an important source of information. For a detailed description of the early safety of SES implantation for patients with acute coronary syndromes, the reader is referred to Chapter 4.

Patient population

From April 2002 to January 2003 (9-month enrolment), a total of 186 consecutive patients with ST-elevation acute myocardial infarction have been treated with primary angioplasty utilizing exclusively sirolimus-eluting stents and are analyzed in this chapter. A control group for comparison was composed of 183 consecutive patients with ST-elevation acute myocardial infarction treated with conventional bare stents in the period immediately prior to the introduction of sirolimus-eluting stents. The following bare metal stents were used: BX Sonic or BX Velocity in 53% (Cordis, a Johnson & Johnson company, Warren, New Jersey), Multi-Link Penta in 22% (Guidant Corp., Santa Clara, California), Multi-Link Tetra in 6% (Guidant Corp., Santa Clara, California), R-Stent in 6% (Orbus Medical Technologies, Ft. Lauderdale, Florida), and other stents in 12%. Both groups included patients admitted with cardiogenic shock (defined as persistent systolic blood pressure <90 mm Hg, or the need of vasopressors or intra-aortic balloon pumping required to maintain blood pressure >90 mm Hg with evidence of end-organ failure and elevated left ventricular filling pressures). In addition, an angiographic substudy was carried out for patients treated in the first 6 months after the introduction of SES (patients with both primary angioplasty or rescue procedures after failed thrombolytic therapy were included in the angiographic substudy).

Table 5.1. Baseline and procedural characteristics of patients treated with bare stents or SES implantation. (Reprinted from Lemos et al.[48a] With permission from American College of Cardiology Foundation)

	Bare stents (n=183)	SES (n=186)	P-value
Male, %	79	75	0.4
Age, years±SD	57±12	60±12	0.04
Diabetes, %	12	11	0.9
Current smoking, %	47	46	0.8
Previous myocardial infarction, %	24	14	0.03
Previous angioplasty, %	9	7	0.4
Previous bypass surgery, %	3	2	0.3
Coronary disease			0.3
Single-vessel, %	48	55	
Double-disease, %	29	27	
Triple-vessel, %	24	18	
Cardiogenic shock, %	10	13	0.3
Time from symptom onset to angioplasty, hours±SD	3.0±2.7	3.2±1.9	0.6
Infarct-related vessel			0.3
Right coronary artery, %	30	37	
Left anterior descending, %	57	53	
Left circumflex artery, %	10	8	
Left main coronary artery, %	1	2	
Bypass graft, %	2	–	
TIMI flow baseline			0.7
Grade 0/I, %	73	73	
Grade II, %	15	17	
Grade III, %	13	10	
TIMI flow after angioplasty			0.5
Grade 0/I, %	4	2	
Grade II, %	17	15	
Grade III, %	79	83	
Number of stents±SD	1.7±1.0	1.9±1.2	0.03
IIbIIIa inhibitor, %	56	37	<0.01
Clopidogrel prescription, months±SD	2.1±1.5	3.7±2.1	<0.01
Peak CK, IU/L±SD*	3957±5135	3126±3126	0.1
Peak CK-MB, IU/L±SD†	319±230	296±255	0.5

CK=creatine kinase; SD=standard deviation; SES=sirolimus-eluting stents
* Upper limit of normal 199 U/L
† Upper limit of normal 23 U/L

Baseline and procedural characteristics

Baseline characteristics were similar between both study groups, except by an older age and a lower incidence of previous myocardial infarction in the sirolimus group (Table 5.1). Procedural characteristics differed between both groups in terms of the utilization of glycoprotein IIb/IIIa inhibitors (sirolimus: 37% vs. bare stents: 56%; p<0.01) and the number of stents implanted (sirolimus: 1.9±1.2 vs. bare stents: 1.7±1.0; p=0.03). As defined by the study protocol, the duration of clopidogrel prescription was longer for patients with sirolimus stents (Table 5.1).

Clinical outcomes

There were no significant differences in the 30-day outcomes between patients treated with sirolimus or bare stents (Table 5.2). Stent thrombosis was diagnosed in 3 patients (1.6%) treated with bare stents and was not detected in the SES group (p=0.1) (Table 5.2). At 300 days, there were no differences between both study groups in the incidence of death and death or re-infarction (Table 5.2). However, the incidence of 300-day major adverse events was

Table 5.2. Kaplan–Meier estimates of adverse events at 30 days and at 300 days. (Reprinted from Lemos et al.[48a] With permission from American College of Cardiology Foundation)

	Bare stents (n=183)	SES (n=186)	p-value
30-day outcomes			
Death, %	5.5	5.9	1.0
Death or non-fatal re-infarction, %	7.1	6.5	0.8
Target vessel revascularization, %	4.4	1.1	0.1
Any event, %	10.4	7.5	0.4
Stent thrombosis, %*	1.6	0	0.1
300-day outcomes			
Death, %	8.2	8.3	0.8
Death or non-fatal re-infarction, %	10.4	8.8	0.5
Target vessel revascularization, %	8.2	1.1	<0.01
Any event, %	17.0	9.4	0.02

SES=sirolimus-eluting stents
*Angiographically documented stent thrombosis

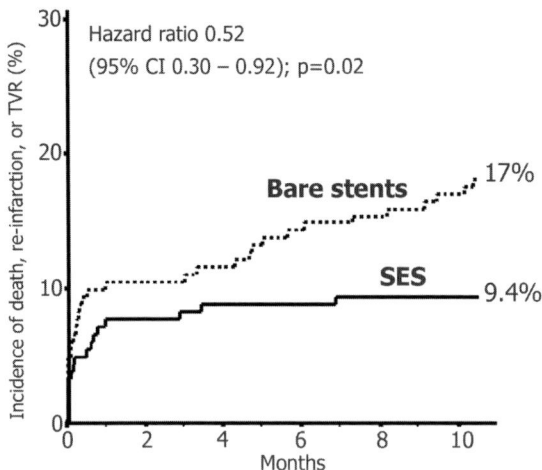

Figure 5.1 Cumulative incidence of death, re-infarction, or target vessel revascularization in patients treated with sirolimus-eluting stents (SES) or bare stents. (Modified from Lemos et al.[48a] With permission from American College of Cardiology Foundation.)

significantly lower in the sirolimus stent group compared to the bare stent group (9.4% vs. 17% respectively; hazard ratio 0.52 [95% confidence interval 0.30–0.92]; p=0.02) (Table 5.2; Figure 5.1), mainly because of a marked reduction in the risk of repeat intervention (1.1% vs. 8.2% respectively; HR 0.21 [95% CI 0.06–0.74]; p=0.01). A multivariate analysis was performed to adjust for baseline and procedural imbalances between the study groups (Table 5.3). Sirolimus-eluting stent utilization was identified as an independent predictor of 300-day death, re-infarction, or repeat revascularization (HR 0.53 [95% CI 0.29–0.95]; p=0.03).

Table 5.3. Multivariate predictors of 300-day major adverse cardiac events. (Reprinted from Lemos et al.[48a] With permission from American College of Cardiology Foundation)

	Hazard ratio	95% confidence interval	p-value
SES utilization	0.53	0.29–0.95	0.03
Cardiogenic shock	3.31	1.72–6.34	<0.01
Culprit vessel left main coronary	6.05	1.60–22.87	<0.01
Culprit vessel left anterior descending	2.02	1.10–3.71	0.02
Post-procedure TIMI flow			<0.01
Grade 0/I (reference)	1.00	–	
Grade II	0.29	0.11–0.76	
Grade III	0.17	0.07–0.40	
Current smoking	0.57	0.31–1.02	0.06

SES=sirolimus-eluting stents
*Angiographically documented stent thrombosis

Table 5.4. Quantitative coronary analysis in patients with acute myocardial infarction treated with sirolimus-eluting stent. (From Saia et al.[48b])

	Pre-procedure	Post-procedure	Follow-up*
Reference diameter, mm	2.73±0.59	2.80±0.47	3.04±0.49
Minimum lumen diameter, mm	0.34±0.50	2.54±1.31	2.59±0.42
Diameter stenosis, %	86±21	14±12	15±11
Lesion length, mm	16.9±9.9	–	–
Late loss, mm	–	–	–0.04±0.25
Binary restenosis, %	–	–	0

* related to 62 patients with 6-month angiographic follow-up

Angiographic outcomes

Six-month angiographic follow-up was obtained from 62 patients treated with SES (70% of eligible patients treated in the period). The angiographic outcomes are shown in Table 5.4. Late loss was –0.04±0.25 mm, and there were no cases of binary restenosis. Figure 5.2 illustrates the baseline, post-procedure, and follow-up angiographies of a typical patient treated with SES in RESEARCH.

Interpretation of the findings

The main findings of the present analysis were that

(1) The risk of subacute thrombosis within the first 30 days did not appear higher compared with bare metal stents;
(2) The incidence of angiographic restenosis after SES implantation for patients with acute myocardial infarction was 'zero', with an almost 'zero' late luminal loss;
(3) Sirolimus-eluting stent implantation was effective in reducing the incidence of adverse events at 300 days in unselected patients with ST-elevation acute myocardial infarction, compared to conventional bare stenting.

Sirolimus-eluting stents were associated with a relative reduction of 48% in the risk of death, re-infarction, or repeat intervention and a relative reduction of 79% in the risk of repeat intervention at 300 days.

45

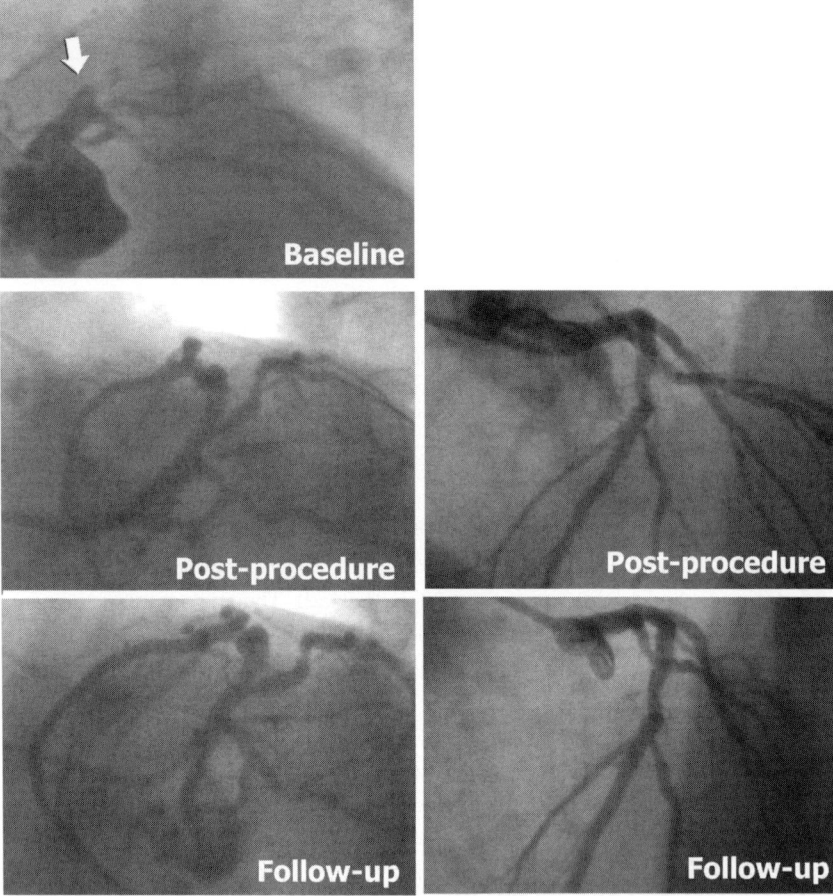

Figure 5.2 Patient admitted for primary recanalization after 3 hours from the onset of an acute myocardial infarction. At the baseline angiogram (upper panel), the left anterior descending artery (LAD) was totally occluded just distal to its origin (arrow). The patient was successfully treated with implantation of a 3 × 18-mm sirolimus-eluting stent at the LAD and balloon dilatation of the ostium of the first diagonal branch (mid panels). At follow-up, the patient was asymptomatic and the coronary angiogram showed no evidence of neo-intimal proliferation.

Reperfusion treatment with sirolimus-eluting stents was associated with similar rates of vessel patency, enzymatic release, and 30-day complications compared to bare stents. The death rate and the incidence of death or re-infarction were similar in both study groups, but somewhat higher than those reported in randomized trials with selected patients.[49,50] These findings most probably reflect the unrestrictive inclusion criteria of the protocol,[51] which frequently enrolled patients not included in randomized studies, like for instance, cardiogenic shock, multivessel disease, and unprotected left main lesions. Importantly, stent thrombosis has not been identified in any patient treated with sirolimus stents and occurred in 3 controls (1.6%), with no statistical difference between the groups. Although the incidence of stent thrombosis in the bare stent group was at a somewhat higher range, the results for this group were not discrepant from historical series with conventional stents.[49,50,52–54]

Coronary stenting for the treatment of acute myocardial infarction has been limited by the need of late repeat intervention, which has been reported to occur in approximately 9% of cases at 6 months, ranging from 3.6% to 22.7%, as shown in Figure 5.3.[49,50,55] The incidence of repeat intervention after conventional stenting in our series (8.2%) was in line with these previous numbers. Conversely, patients treated with sirolimus-eluting stent implantation had clearly a reduced risk of re-intervention at 10 months. Of note, between 30 days and 10 months, no additional patient was referred for repeat

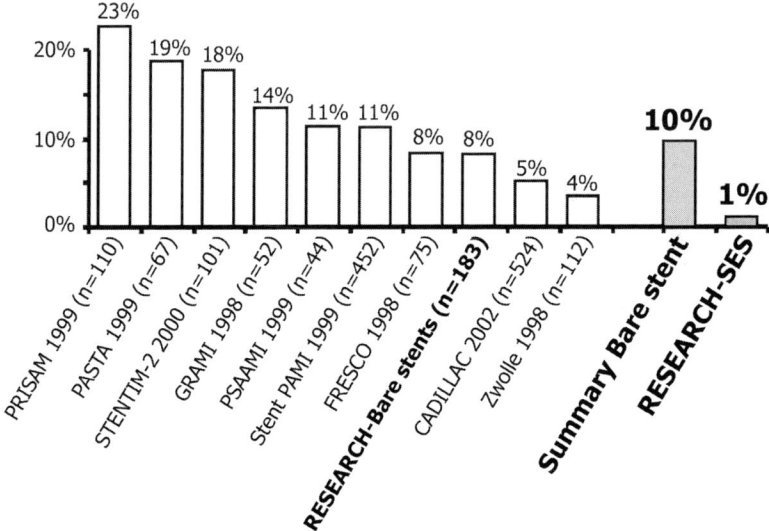

Figure 5.3 Randomized trials for acute myocardial infarction patients evaluating primary angioplasty with balloon angioplasty vs. conventional stents. The figure shows the 6/12-month repeat revascularization in the stent arms of these trials and in the RESEARCH registry (10-month follow-up). The re-intervention rate of patients treated with bare stents in the RESEARCH is in line with that from the previous randomized trials (8% and 10% respectively) and both figures contrast with the markedly lower incidence of re-intervention for SES treated patients.

revascularization, which is consistent with the lack of angiographic restenosis after sirolimus stent implantation.

The peri- and post-procedural antiplatelet therapeutic scheme differed between patients treated with bare or sirolimus stents in our series. Patients in the sirolimus group received less glycoprotein IIb/IIIa inhibitors but had a longer clopidogrel prescription time. However, none of these characteristics were identified as independent predictors influencing the outcomes of patients. The impact of clopidogrel and glycoprotein IIb/IIIa inhibitors on the long-term clinical outcomes of patients with ST elevation acute myocardial infarction still remain to be established.[49,56,57]

In conclusion, sirolimus-eluting stent implantation for unselected patients with ST elevation acute myocardial infarction was associated with similar procedural and 30-days outcomes compared to bare stents, but markedly reduced the risk of major adverse events and repeat intervention at 10 months owing to a 'zero' incidence of restenosis. By providing effective mechanical reperfusion with similar results to the current therapeutic standard, and decreasing the incidence of late complications, sirolimus-eluting stents appeared as an attractive approach for patients admitted with acute myocardial infarction.

6. Sirolimus-Eluting Stents for Patients with Impaired Renal Function

Pedro A Lemos, Ron T van Domburg, Patrick W Serruys

Introduction

Chronic kidney disease is increasingly being recognized as an important risk factor for future adverse events in patients with coronary disease.[58–71] Moreover, the importance of kidney dysfunction is further maximized by its rising prevalence, which is expected to more than double in the next decade.[70] The treatment of coronary heart disease in patients with renal impairment is often complicated by the presence of multiple co-morbidities and limitations in drug prescription.

The present chapter evaluates the impact of baseline renal function on the 1-year mortality and repeat intervention of patients treated with either conventional bare stents or sirolimus-eluting stents (SES).

Patient population and renal function evaluation

From October 2001 until October 2002 (6-month enrolment for both the pre-sirolimus and the sirolimus phases), a total of 1262 consecutive non-dialysis patients were treated with bare stents or sirolimus eluting-stents in the 2 study periods. From these, 1080 patients (86%) had pre-procedure serum creatinine measured in our institution and compose the present study population (bare stent group=543 patients; sirolimus-eluting stent group=537 patients).

The closest creatinine values before the procedure were used to calculate baseline creatinine clearance according to the Cockcroft and Gault formula.[72] Renal impairment was defined as a calculated creatinine clearance below 60 ml/min, a cutoff value previously proposed by the National Kidney Foundation–Kidney Disease Outcome Quality Initiative Advisory Board to identify patients with moderate renal impairment[68] and the American Heart

Association Councils on Kidney in Cardiovascular Disease, High Blood Pressure Research, Clinical Cardiology, and Epidemiology and Prevention.[70]

Baseline and procedural characteristics

In the bare stent group (n=543), 92 patients (17%) had renal dysfunction. Similarly, in the SES group (n=537), 94 patients (18%) had renal dysfunction. The mean creatinine clearance was 49 ml/min in patients with renal impairment and was 100 ml/min in patients with normal renal function (p<0.01); the average serum creatinine was 1.3 mg/dl in patients with renal dysfunction and 0.9 mg/dl in patients with normal renal function. Patients with renal impairment were older (72±8 years vs. 59±10 years; p<0.01) and more frequently female (49% vs. 76%; p<0.01). They had more hypertension (49% vs. 49%; p<0.01), previous coronary surgery (23% vs. 8%; p<0.01), triple-vessel disease (35% vs. 17%; p<0.01), bypass graft stenting (12% vs. 3%; p<0.01), and a higher number of stents implanted per procedure (2.3 vs. 2.0; p<0.01). The average creatinine clearance was similar between patients treated with sirolimus or bare stents.

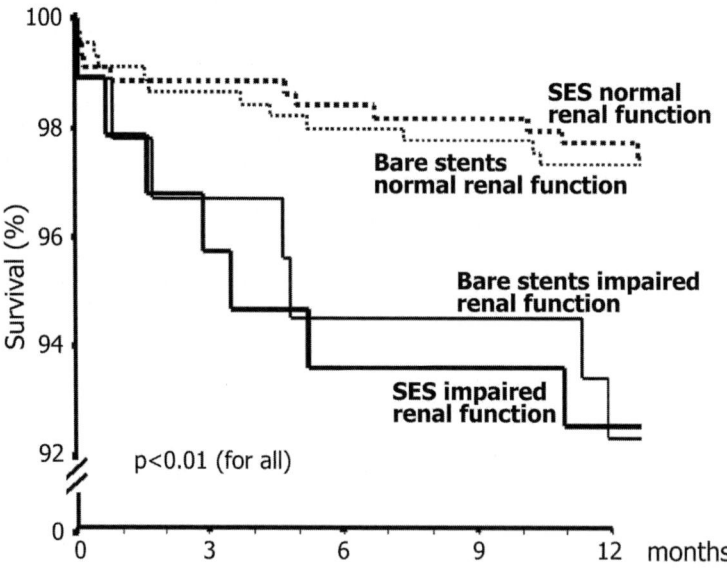

Figure 6.1 One-year mortality after sirolimus-eluting stent (SES) implantation or bare stent implantation for patients with or without renal impairment. Note that, overall, patients with renal impairment have a significantly higher risk of death than patients normal renal function. However, in both renal function groups, the incidence of death is virtually the same between patients treated with SES or bare stent.

One-year outcomes

The median follow-up period was 421 days (interquartile range: 391–459 days). The 1-year mortality rate was significantly higher in patients with renal impairment than in patients with normal renal function (both stent types analyzed together) (7.6% vs. 2.5% respectively; hazard ratio 3.14 [95% CI: 1.68–5.88]; p<0.01). Similarly, when analyzed separately, baseline renal impairment significantly increased the risk of death in patients treated with

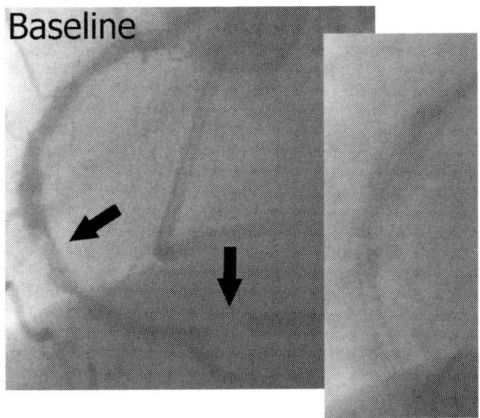

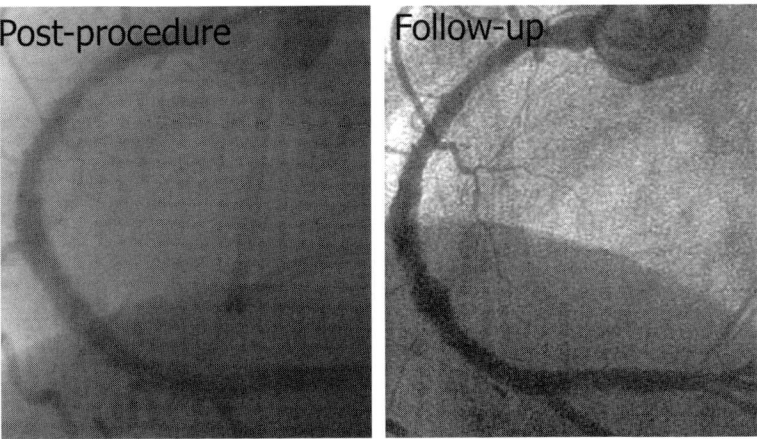

Figure 6.2 *Patient with renal failure presenting with stable angina. At baseline, two stenosis were detected in the mid and distal portions of the right coronary artery (top arrows), with severe angiographic calcification (top, detail). The patient was treated with implantation of two, non-overlapping, sirolimus-eluting stents (both 3 × 18 mm), with good final angiographic result (bottom left) that was maintained at 6-month re-evaluation (bottom right).*

either bare stents or sirolimus-eluting stents. Moreover, the negative effect of renal impairment on mortality was similar between patients treated with bare stent and SES (Figure 6.1). Importantly, when compared to bare stents, SES were effective in reducing the risk of target vessel revascularization both in patients without (unadjusted hazard ratio 0.59; [95% CI 0.39–0.90]; p=0.01) and in patients with renal impairment (unadjusted hazard ratio 0.37; [95% CI 0.15–0.90]; p=0.03) (Figure 6.2).

Interpretation of the findings

Neither surgical nor percutaneous revascularization have been shown to eliminate the increased risk of patients with renal impairment.[61–63,66,67,69] Patients with renal failure have a higher mortality after successful percutaneous coronary intervention.[61,62,67] It has been previously questioned whether the occurrence of restenosis contributes to the increased risk of death in these patients.[61,67] This chapter shows that impaired renal function significantly increases 1-year mortality after percutaneous coronary revascularization, regardless of the use of sirolimus-eluting stents or conventional bare stents. In spite of presenting a clear anti-restenotic effect, sirolimus-eluting stents were not associated with decreased mortality rates in patients with renal dysfunction. The findings in the present chapter, therefore, challenge the concept that the increased mortality of patients with renal impairment is attributable to the occurrence of restenosis. Nevertheless, even though the mortality risk was not decreased in the present series, the marked reduction of repeat revascularization with sirolimus-eluting stents represents an important therapeutic achievement for patients with renal impairment.

7. SIROLIMUS-ELUTING STENTS FOR PATIENTS WITH PRIOR CORONARY BYPASS GRAFT SURGERY

Angela Hoye, Patrick W Serruys

Introduction

Recurrence of ischemia and angina after coronary artery bypass graft surgery (CABG) relates to either progression of native vessel atherosclerosis or failure of the bypass grafts themselves. Indeed, angiographic studies have shown that by 10–12 years, 75–79% vein grafts are occluded or severely diseased.[73,74] Moreover, it has been also shown that the bypass operation may accelerate disease progression within the native vessels.[75,76] Therefore, recurrence of anginal symptoms occurs relatively frequently following CABG,[77] a condition that may lead to the need for further revascularization. However, repeat CABG surgery is associated with a higher mortality rates compared to a first operation.[78,79] In this context, percutaneous revascularization may be an attractive therapeutic strategy. Unfortunately, stent implantation in venous bypass grafts carries a high subsequent rate of restenosis of 37–53%.[80,81] Furthermore, lesions located at the native coronary bed of patients with prior CABG frequently carry a high risk of restenosis, because of the common frequency of chronic total occlusions and lesions located at peripheral segments with a small caliber, among others reasons. This chapter analyses the impact of sirolimus-eluting stents for patients with previous CABG treated in RESEARCH.

Patient population and procedural data

The current study cohort comprises of 47 patients with a previous history of CABG who were treated for *de novo* lesions solely with SES. A control group (n=66) comprised of patients who had been treated similarly in the preceding 6 months though with bare stents.

Baseline patient demographics and procedural data are presented in Table 7.1. There were no significant differences between the 2 groups treated with

Table 7.1: Baseline patient demographics. (From Hoye et al.[81a])

	Bare stent n=66	SES group n=47	p value
Male sex (%)	66.7	70.3	0.5
Mean age (years)	69±11	68±9	1.0
Current smoker (%)	16.7	10.6	0.4
Diabetes mellitus (%)	19.7	21.3	1.0
Previous MI (%)	47.7	31.9	0.2
Previous PCI (%)	39.4	42.6	0.9
Multivessel disease (%)	95.5	91.5	0.5
Clinical presentation			0.2
Stable angina (%)	48.5	63.8	
Unstable angina (%)	43.9	34.0	
Acute MI (%)	7.6	2.1	
GP IIb/IIIa inhibitor	36.4	21.3	0.1
Treated vessel			
Left anterior descending (%)	34.8	42.6	0.4
Left circumflex (%)	33.3	29.8	0.8
Right coronary artery (%)	27.3	17.0	0.3
Left main coronary (%)	15.2	10.6	0.6
Bypass graft (%)	40.9	36.2	0.7
Mean number of stents	2.1±1.4	1.9±0.9	0.7
Mean stent diameter (mm)	3.3±0.6	2.8±0.3	<0.01
Stented length per patient (mm)	35.1±24.7	32.6±22.1	1.0
Angiographic success (%)	98.5	97.9	1.0

either bare stents or SES, except in the mean nominal diameter of the stent utilized, which was smaller in the SES group. Intervention within native coronary arteries only, occurred in 59.9% of the bare stent group, and 63.8% of the SES group. The angiographic success rate in both groups was high at >97%. Table 7.2 presents the Kaplan–Meier estimates of the major adverse cardiac events of the two groups at 1 year. There is a significantly lower rate of events in the SES group, which is predominantly related to a reduced need for repeat target vessel revascularization (Table 7.2; Figure 7.1). Two clinical cases are illustrated in Figures 7.2 and 7.3.

Interpretation of the findings

Previous data show that percutaneous intervention with bare stents in patients with a history of previous CABG, is associated with an increased rate of MACE compared to those without prior CABG.[82–87] This relates, at least in part, to

Table 7.2: Kaplan-Meier estimates of 1–year major adverse events. (From Hoye et al.[81a])

	Bare stents	SES	HR	95% CI	p-value
Survival, %	93.9	97.9	0.34	0.04–3.09	0.3
Survival free of myocardial infarction, %	89.4	93.6	0.80	0.24–2.71	0.7
Survival free of myocardial infarction or target vessel revascularization, %	69.7	91.5	0.37	0.15–0.91	0.03

the association of this group of patients with an adverse risk profile as patients tend to be older, and have a higher prevalence of diabetes, and multivessel disease.[82–87] Moreover, this increase in MACE is evident whether patients are being treated in the context of either stable angina, or an acute coronary syndrome.[82–87] However, this chapter demonstrates that utilization of the sirolimus-eluting stent for patients with previous CABG significantly reduces the rate of major adverse cardiac events (MACE) compared to those treated with bare metal stents.

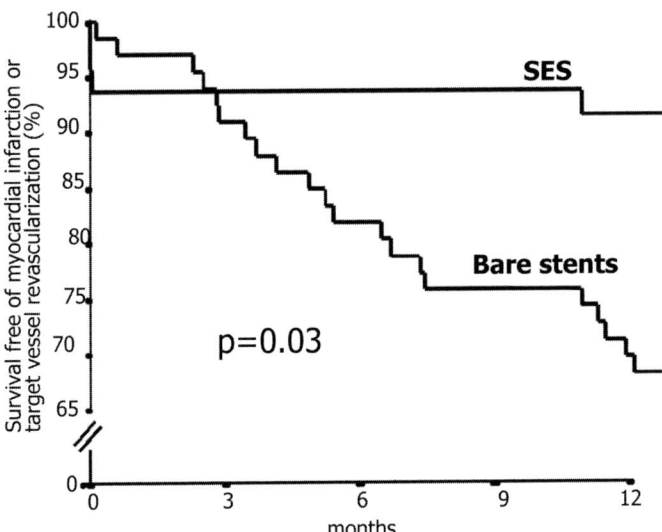

Figure 7.1 Survival free of myocardial infarction or target vessel revascularization in patients with previous CABG treated with sirolimus-eluting stents (SES) or bare stents. (From Hoye et al.[81a])

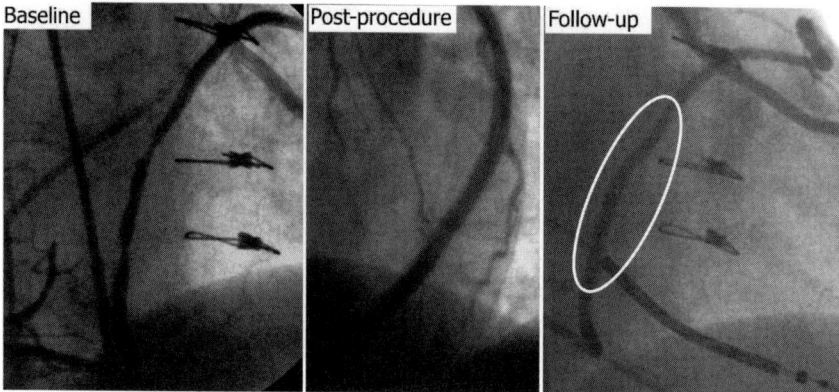

Figure 7.2 Patient with previous coronary surgery showing a diseased saphenous vein graft with two tandem stenoses (left panel). Two overlapping sirolimus-eluting stents (3.0 × 33 mm and 3.0 × 18 mm) were implanted over the diseased segment, with post-dilatation of with a 3.5-mm balloon (mid panel). At 6-month follow-up, the patient was asymptomatic with no evidence of neointimal proliferation inside the stents or at the stent borders (right).

It is 20 years since Douglas et al demonstrated the feasibility of PCI in patients with a history of CABG.[88] More recently, the AWESOME randomized trial and registry demonstrated that at three years, the overall survival of patients with previous CABG and medically refractory angina, was similar whether treated with either PCI or re-do CABG.[89] Moreover, when given the choice of PCI or re-do CABG, the majority of patients preferred the former option. The investigators concluded that PCI might be the preferred revascularization strategy. In the RESEARCH population presented in this chapter, 40.9% in the bare stent group, and 36.2% of the SES group underwent intervention with at least one bypass graft. Compared to native vessels, percutaneous revascularization of diseased saphenous vein grafts is hampered by an increased rate of adverse events, thereby contributing to the worse outcome of post-CABG patients. Procedural complications may relate to distal embolization of friable material within the graft, and at follow-up, grafts are subject to an increased rate of restenosis. Historically, results of balloon-only therapy were disappointing.[90–92] In one study of 454 patients, procedural success was 90%, with a 5-year MACE-free survival of only 26%.[93] Subsequently, a randomized trial demonstrated the benefit of stenting over balloon angioplasty. At 6-months, the rate of survival free from either death, myocardial infarction, repeat CABG, or target lesion revascularization (TLR) was 73% in the stented group versus just 58% in the balloon-only group

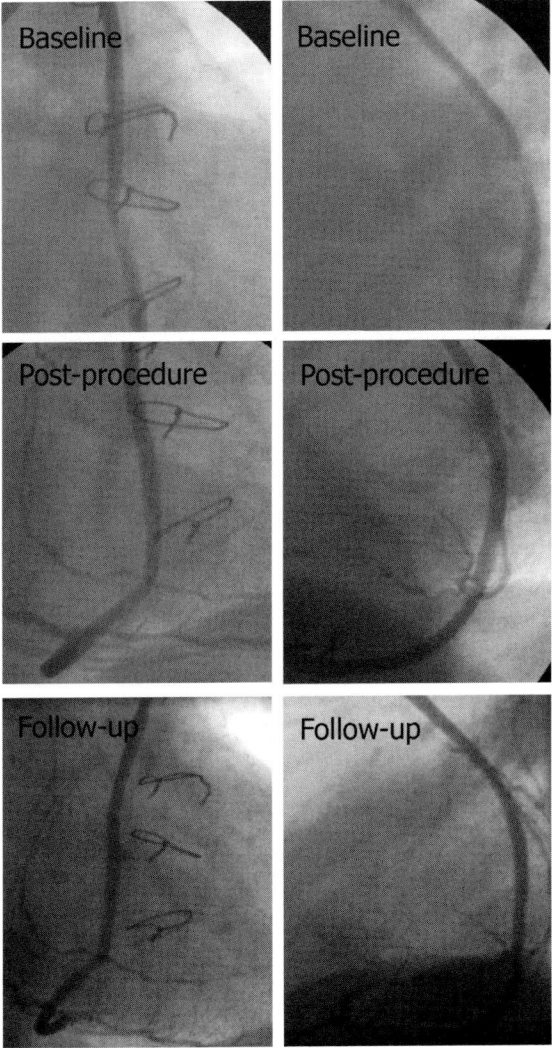

Figure 7.3 *Discrete luminal stenosis in the shaft of a saphenous vein graft (upper panels) treated with a sirolimus-eluting stent (mid panel). At angiographic follow-up, no neointimal re-narrowing was noted at the stented segment (lower panels).*

(p=0.03).[80] However, the angiographic restenosis rate remained high (37% versus 46% respectively, p=0.24).

The major limitation of PCI has always been the development of in-stent restenosis and subsequent need for repeat revascularization. In particular, restenosis rates utilizing bare stents within saphenous venous bypass grafts range between 37–53%.[80,81] Intervention solely within native vessels was undertaken in 59.9% of the bare stent group, and 63.8% of the SES group.

The type of native vessel disease manifested in a population with a history of previous CABG can be difficult to effectively treat percutaneously; lesions may be ostial, or chronically occluded, or the disease may be diffuse and the arteries small and calcified. These features, together with the increased prevalence of diabetes in these patients, tend to increase the risk of developing restenosis.[92,94]

In summary, in the present chapter it was observed that sirolimus-eluting stents reduces the subsequent rate of adverse events at one year, in a high risk population with a history of previous coronary artery bypass graft surgery.

8. SIROLIMUS-ELUTING STENTS FOR LEFT MAIN CORONARY ARTERY DISEASE

Chourmouzios A Arampatzis, Patrick W Serruys

Introduction

Several trials have reported on the safety and feasibility of stent implantation to treat left main (LM) coronary disease, with favorable procedural and long-term results.[95–98] However, restenosis remains the major complication limiting late outcome after percutaneous intervention. In patients treated with LM stenting, the occurrence of restenosis has been particularly associated with hazardous clinical manifestations.[99] In this viewpoint, although percutaneous intervention has increasingly been reported as a possible therapeutic alternative, surgical revascularization remains the most appropriate therapy.[100] In this chapter, the efficacy of the sirolimus-eluting stent (SES) for patients treated for LM disease is evaluated.

Patient population and procedural characteristics

In the current chapter, 30 patients treated for LM artery disease in the first 6 months of the RESEARCH are described. Patients enrolled in this study were divided into 3 groups: (1) 5 patients treated within the acute phase of myocardial infarction; (2) 9 patients with bailout stenting for LM dissection that occurred during angioplasty (4 had dissection induced by the guiding catheter, 1 due to wire exit, and 3 due to proximal left anterior descending stenting) or during conventional diagnostic procedures (1 patient); (3) 16 elective patients with *de novo* lesions. The subset of elective patients with *de novo* LM lesions (n=16) were analyzed separately, with a more prolonged follow-up period and late angiographic re-study. Protected LM segment was defined by the presence of a patent coronary artery bypass graft. LM dilatation was performed with implantation of a 3.0-mm SES in all patients (largest diameter available at the time of this study).

Table 8.1. Baseline clinical and procedural characteristics (n=30)

	Acute myocardial infarction (n=5)	Bail out stenting (n=9)	Elective (n=16)
Age (years)	64±9	65±16	65±11
Men	3 (60%)	4 (45%)	11 (69%)
Hypercholesterolemia	3 (60%)	5 (56%)	4 (25%)
Treated diabetes mellitus	1 (20%)	3 (33%)	7 (44%)
Treated systemic hypertension	0 (0%)	3 (33%)	2 (13%)
Prior myocardial infarction	0 (0%)	3 (33%)	5 (31%)
Prior angioplasty	0 (0%)	2 (22%)	5 (31%)
Clinical presentation			
Stable angina pectoris	-	6 (67%)	16 (100%)
Unstable angina	-	3 (33%)	0 (0%)
Lesion location			
Ostial	2 (40%)	6 (67%)	5 (31%)
Body	2 (40%)	0 (0%)	1 (6%)
Bifurcation	1 (20%)	3 (33%)	10 (63%)
Stents per patient	3±2.3	4.5±1.9	2.9±1.6
Direct stenting	3 (60%)	9 (100%)	5 (29%)
IIb/IIIa inhibitors	4 (80%)	5 (56%)	5 (31%)
Cardiogenic shock	4 (80%)	0 (0%)	0 (0%)
Hemodynamic assist			
Intra aortic balloon	4 (80%)	1 (11%)	0 (0%)
Left ventricle assist device	0 (0%)	0 (0%)	3 (18%)

Baseline clinical and procedural characteristics of the study group are listed in Table 8.1. Overall, unprotected LM disease was present in 65% (9 patients [56%] in the elective subgroup had an unprotected left main). Four patients with acute myocardial infarction were admitted with cardiogenic shock (80%). Intra-aortic balloon pump or left ventricular assistance devices were used in patients with either hemodynamic compromise (n=5) or in elective patients deemed to have a very high procedural risk (n=3).[101] Postdilatation after SES deployment (with 3.5-mm to 4.5-mm balloons) was performed in 23 patients (77%). The distal LM bifurcation was treated in 14 patients (47%); in these patients, both the parent and side branch vessels received a SES.

Clinical outcomes

Table 8.2 lists the clinical outcomes for patients with acute myocardial infarction, bailout stenting, and elective angioplasty. The incidence of

Table 8.2. In-hospital events (n=30)

	Acute MI (n=5)	Bailout stenting (n=9)	Elective (n=16)
Deaths	3 (60%)	1 (11%)	0 (0%)
Myocardial Infarction	0 (0%)	0 (0%)	1 (6%)
Percutaneous revascularization	0 (0%)	0 (0%)	0 (0%)
Coronary bypass	0 (0%)	1 (11%)	0 (0%)
Major cardiac events	3 (60%)	2 (22%)	1 (6%)

in-hospital major cardiac events was 60%, 22%, and 6% in the 3 groups, respectively. The in-hospital mortality rate in patients with acute myocardial infarction was 60%, in the bailout group 11%, and in elective patients, the rate was 0%. All 3 deaths in the acute myocardial infarction group occurred in patients admitted in cardiogenic shock (2 presented with a totally occluded LM segment). In-hospital repeat revascularization occurred in only 1 patient. This patient had been successfully treated for LM dissection, but developed cardiac tamponade after the procedure and underwent surgical pericardial drainage, during which time he received a venous graft to the first obtuse marginal branch.

Postdischarge complete clinical follow-up is reported in Table 8.3 and was available for all living patients, except for 1 patient (who could not be contacted). Mean follow-up was 5 months for the bailout and acute MI subgroups. There were no postdischarge deaths, myocardial infarctions, or percutaneous revascularizations in these subgroups. One patient underwent elective minimally invasive coronary bypass (total target vessel revascularization rate of 4%). Initially, this patient had an SES implantation for iatrogenic dissection of the LM segment. This patient's nontreated vessel (chronic, totally

Table 8.3. Post-discharge events (in-hospital events are excluded) for the Acute MI and Bailout Stenting Subgroups (mean follow-up 5 months, n=10)

	Acute MI (n=2)	Bailout stenting (n=8)
Deaths	0 (0%)	0 (0%)
Myocardial infarction	0 (0%)	0 (0%)
Percutaneous revascularization	0 (0%)	0 (0%)
Coronary bypass	0 (0%)	1 (12%)
Major cardiac events	0 (0%)	1 (12%)

61

Table 8.4. One-year clinical outcome for patients treated electively for LM disease

	Late outcome
Deaths, %	0
Myocardial infarction, %	1 (6%)
Reintervention	
Percutaneous revascularization	1 (6%)
Coronary bypass	0
Cumulative incidence of MACE*	2 (12%)
*MACE=major adverse cardiac events	

occluded left anterior descending artery) underwent elective revascularization 1 month later.

Elective patients were followed-up for an average of 12 months (Table 8.4). There were no cases of acute, subacute or late thrombosis, or death. One patient required TLR, for proximal edge restenosis. This patient was a diabetic male, with LM ostial stenosis protected by a patent left internal mammary artery. The stenosis was very heavily calcified as indicated by the fact that the cutting balloon ruptured, and was stented with a 3 × 18 mm and 3 × 8 mm SES. Post dilatation was done with a 4.0 mm balloon and the post-procedure diameter stenosis was 43%. Follow-up intracoronary ultrasound revealed underexpansion of the stent, which was due to severe calcification at the ostium. Six-month angiographic follow-up was obtained in 12 patients (75%) of elective patients (Table 8.5). The late lumen loss was 0.04±0.65 mm. There was one patient with restenosis, which represents an 8% angiographic restenosis rate at 1 year. Figures 8.1 and 8.2 illustrate two cases of patients

Table 8.5. Quantitative coronary angiography for patients treated electively for LM disease (n=12 [75% of the initial population]). Catheterization and Cardiovascular Interventions. © 2004

	Index procedure		Follow-up
	Pre	Post	
Reference diameter, mm±SD	2.92±0.66	3.45±0.66	3.24±0.57
Minimum luminal diameter, mm±SD	1.19±0.49	2.83±0.73	2.97±0.66
Acute gain, mm±SD		1.65±0.43	
Late loss, mm±SD			0.04±0.65
Restenosis rate, %			1 (8%)

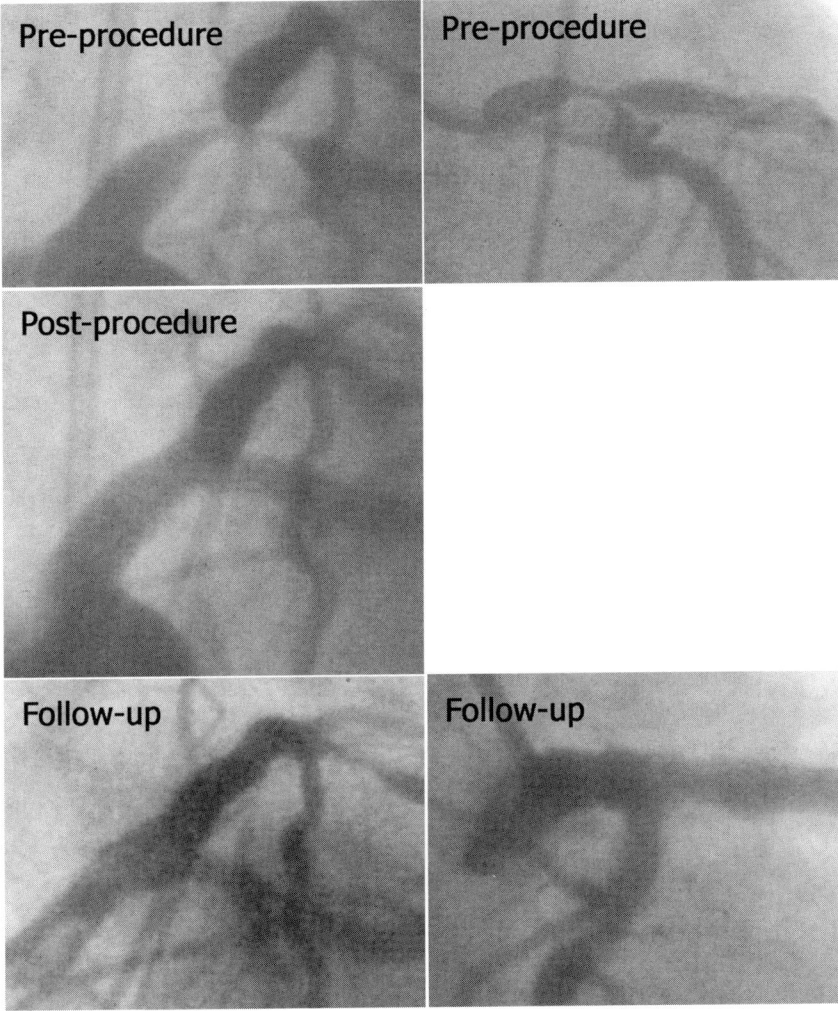

Figure 8.1 Forty seven-year old female with end-stage renal failure, non-insulin-dependent diabetes, hypertension, and hepatitis B virus infection, admitted with stable angina. The upper panels show the baseline coronary angiogram with a severe stenosis in the distal left main coronary involving ostia of the left anterior descending and left circumflex arteries. Surgical treatment was refused due to associated co-morbidities. The patient was treated with elective implantation of two sirolimus eluting-stents (3 × 18-mm and 3 × 33-mm) at the left main bifurcation ('T' stenting technique) with kissing balloon post-dilatation. The mid panel shows the final angiographic result. At 6 months, the patient was asymptomatic and the follow-up angiogram showed widely patent sirolimus-eluting stents (lower panels).

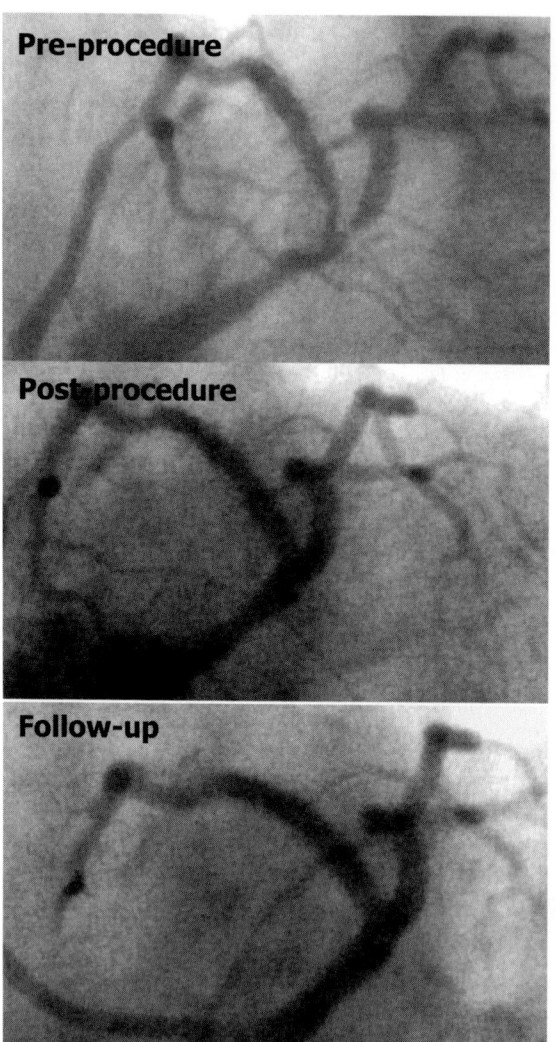

Figure 8.2 Seventy-nine year old male admitted with rest unstable angina. A diagnostic angiogram (upper panel) showed narrowing of the distal left main coronary (LMC) with tight stenosis at the left anterior descending (LAD) and left circumflex (LCx) arteries ostia. The patient was treated with successful implantation of two SES (LMC-LAD 3.0 × 18-mm and LCx 3.0 × 8-mm), shown in the mid panel. After 1 year, the patient underwent angiographic re-study due to atypical chest complaints (lower panel) that showed absence of neointimal proliferation. The patient was kept on medical therapy.

receiving sirolimus-eluting stents for left main disease who underwent late angiographic follow-up.

Interpretation of the findings

Recently, several studies have demonstrated that stenting of the LM artery may be a safe and effective alternative to the surgical approach in carefully selected patients.[95–97] Although the in-hospital success rates are extremely acceptable, the death rate increases gradually within 6 months after the index procedure, and thereafter reoccurrence of major cardiac events is mainly attributed to progression of atherosclerosis.[99] Solving restenosis apparently is the key to improving the long-term outcome in these patients.

The extremely high in-house mortality rate in the myocardial infarction group mirrors the fatal risk of patients having LM disease in this clinical scenario. The findings presented in this chapter agree with previous studies reporting in-hospital mortality rates of acute myocardial infarction due to LM lesions of 55% to 80%.[102,103] The major finding of this report is the absence of fatal events in all patients discharged from the hospital; this study highlights the outstanding performance of the SES. The low rate of percutaneous reintervention after discharge in the overall group and the low rate of angiographic restenosis in the elective subgroup reinforce the efficacy of the SES.

High-pressure post-dilatations with larger balloons were used to optimize stent-to-wall apposition, and overcome the 3-mm width availability of the SES. It is not known whether this (sometimes extreme) postdilatation will affect the elution properties and compromise the polymer's performance (the reader is referred to Chapters 3 and 16). Furthermore, by spreading the struts widely apart, the amount of drug per square millimeter of artery may be reduced and thus impair the efficacy of the SES. However, in the RESEARCH subgroup presented in this chapter, the rate of out-of-hospital clinical events was extremely low. Thus, the discrepancy between stent and postdilatation balloon size does not appear to be of clinical significance.

9. SIROLIMUS-ELUTING STENTS FOR PATIENTS WITH MULTIVESSEL CORONARY DISEASE

Chourmouzios A Arampatzis, Pedro A Lemos

Introduction

The treatment of multivessel disease with percutaneous techniques has been limited by the need for repeat revascularization.[54,104–108] Multiple lesion stenting may importantly increase the chance of restenosis on a per-patient basis.[109] Moreover, patients with multivessel disease and concomitant left anterior descending (LAD) artery stenosis may be particularly prone to need a repeat intervention.[110] In face of this, surgical treatment is frequently chosen as the best therapeutic option for patients with more advanced forms of coronary heart disease. This chapter, therefore, examines the impact of SES for patients with multivessel stenoses and LAD involvement treated in RESEARCH.

Patient population

The population presented in this chapter is composed of 99 consecutive patients (first 6 months of the RESEARCH) without previous bypass surgery who were treated electively with SES implantation in the left anterior descending (LAD) territory, together with stenting in the left circumflex (LCx) and/or right coronary artery (RCA) territories (i.e. revascularization of multivessel stenoses involving the LAD). Routinely, in RESEARCH, an experienced interventional cardiologist and a cardiothoracic surgeon discuss all patients referred for revascularization. When both agree on equivalence of revascularization, then the patient is treated percutaneously in the first instance. Baseline and procedural characteristics are depicted in Table 9.1. Mean age was 64±11 years, 42 patients (42%) were treated for unstable angina, diabetes was present in 25 patients (25%), and 31 (31%) had previous myocardial infarction.

Table 9.1. Baseline and procedural characteristics in 99 patients treated with SES for multivessel disease involving the LAD

Age, years±SD	64±11
Male, %	66
Treated diabetes, %	25
Treated hypertension, %	51
Treated hypercholesterolemia, %	68
Current smoking, %	24
Previous MI, %	31
Previous PCI, %	19
Stable angina, %	58
Unstable angina, %	42
LCx treated (including LAD), %	52
RCA treated (including LAD), %	32
Triple vessel treatment, %	16
Glycoprotein IIbIIIa inhibitor, %	25
ACC/AHA lesion type*, n=293 lesions	
Type A, B1, %	38
Type B2, C, %	62
Number of implanted stents per patient±SD	3.5±1.5
Total stented length per patient,±SD	62.6±32.1
Nominal stent diameter utilized, mm±SD	2.6±0.3

LAD=left anterior descending, MI=myocardial infarction, LCx=left circumflex, RCA=right coronary artery

Procedural characteristics

Overall, 15 patients (15%) were treated for at least one chronic total occlusion (> 3-month duration) and 5 patients (5%) with in-stent restenosis. As described above, all patients received SES in the LAD. Among the 99 patients treated, 46 (46%) received SES in the proximal LAD, 56 (56%) in the middle LAD, 7 (7%) in the distal and 24 (24%) were treated in any of the

Table 9.2. 12-month Kaplan–Meier estimates of adverse events for patients with multivessel disease involving the LAD treated with SES.

Survival, %	99.0%
Survival free of myocardial infarction, %	96.9%
Survival free of myocardial infarction or repeat revascularization, % †	85.6%

* non-Q wave myocardial infarction [peaked creatine kinase 567 U/l (MB fraction: 62 U/l)].
† includes all repeat revascularization in any epicardial vessel

diagonal branches. Additional SES stenting was undertaken in the RCA, LCx, and in both vessels 32 (32%), 51 (52%), 16 (16%) respectively. Overall, 295 lesions were treated (2.9±1.1 lesions per patient) with a mean stent utilization of 3.5±1.5 per patient; a total of 20 patients (20%), received more than 5 stents.

Clinical outcomes

Clinical outcomes at 12 months are presented in Table 9.2. Overall 8 patients (8%) required subsequent revascularization. Among these, 4 patients (4%) had TLR. Two patients, originally treated for chronic total occlusion, had focal in-stent restenosis in the overlapping segment of two SES. The third had an underexpanded stent at the ostium of the RCA (which was heavily calcified) and had additional cutting balloon dilatation. The fourth patient had a TLR due to restenosis at the proximal edge of the SES. A further 4 patients (4%) had percutaneous reintervention in an untreated segment due to progression of atherosclerosis. There were no cases of acute or subacute thrombosis (angiographically documented stent thrombosis requiring repeat intervention). After 12 months, the survival rate free of events at one year was 85.6%. Figure 9.1 shows an illustrative case of multivessel treatment with SES.

Interpretation of the findings

Patients treated with SES in a scenario of multivessel stenting, involving the LAD had a low incidence of adverse events, with remarkably low rates of repeat revascularization; the freedom from revascularization was 92% at one year. For comparison, patients treated with conventional stenting in the randomized Arterial Revascularization Therapy Study (ARTS), Argentine Randomized Study: Coronary Angioplasty with Stenting versus Coronary Bypass Surgery in patients with Multiple-Vessel Disease (ERACI II), and Stent or Surgery (SOS) trials had freedom from revascularization rates of 79%, 83.2% and 79% respectively.[54,105,108] The survival free of any event in the present series was 85.6%, which appears to be distinctly better than that observed in the stent arm of ARTS (73.8%). Actually, the present findings with SES closely resembled the survival free of adverse events seen in its surgical arm of ARTS (85.6% and 87.8% respectively). Figure 9.2 shows the Kaplan–Meier curve for survival free of adverse events of the present series.

69

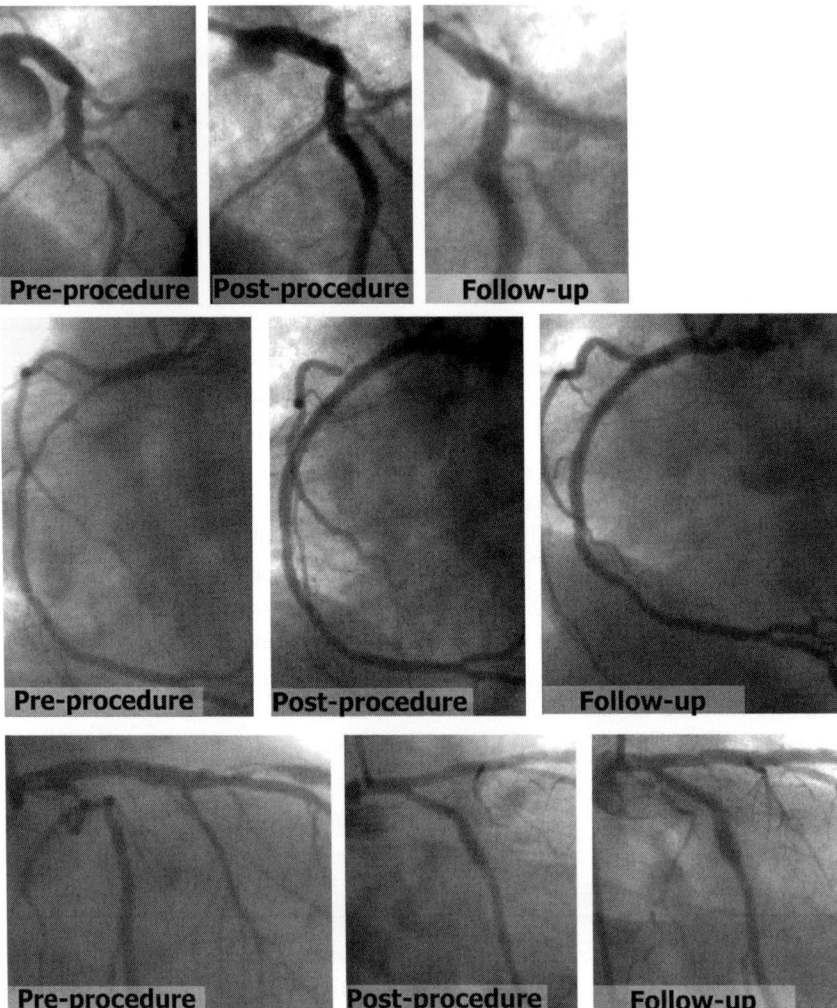

Figure 9.1 *Triple-vessel sirolimus-eluting stent (SES) implantation in a 40-year-old patient admitted with unstable angina. The patient presented a discrete lesion in the proximal left anterior descending artery treated with one 3.0 × 18-mm SES (upper panel). A long coronary lesion was also detected in the proximal-mid right coronary artery and was treated with a 3 × 33-mm SES (mid panel). Moreover, the left circumflex artery presented a tight luminal narrowing at its proximal portion, which was treated with the implantation of three SES, due to border dissection after implantation of the first stent. After 7 months, the patient was asymptomatic and showed widely patent stented segments, with no evidence of neointimal proliferation at late angiographic examination.*

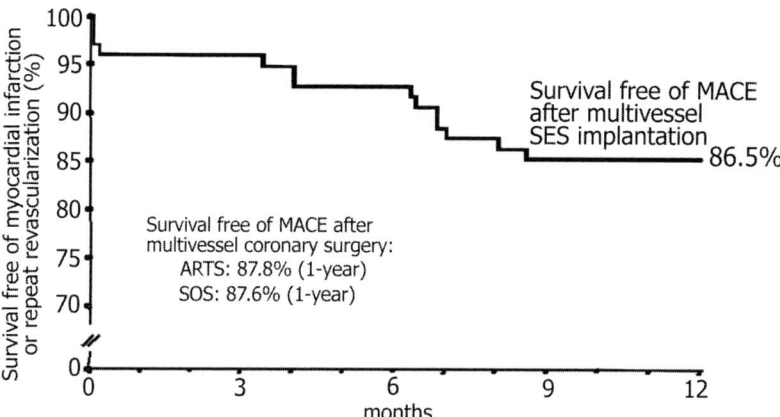

Figure 9.2 *Kaplan–Meier curves for the survival free of myocardial infarction or repeat revascularization of 99 patients treated with SES for multivessel disease and LAD involvement. Also, the rates of survival free of adverse events of the surgical arm of the ARTS[54] and SOS[108] trials are depicted.*

Also, the rates of survival free of adverse events of the surgical arm of the ARTS[54] and SOS[108] trials are depicted. Interestingly, the survival free of major events after multivessel SES implantation seen in the present chapter and the findings observed after surgical treatment in those trials were very similar. Obviously, no formal comparison can be done between the different studies. Nevertheless, the potential benefit of SES is readily suggested by the present results, which implies the promising role of SES for the treatment of patients with multivessel disease.

In conclusion, sirolimus-eluting stent implantation for patients with multivessel disease involving the LAD is associated with low incidence of adverse events at one year, particularly of subsequent revascularization. Multilesion SES implantation is a promising therapeutic strategy for patients with advanced coronary artery disease.

10. SIROLIMUS-ELUTING STENTS FOR ELDERLY PATIENTS

Maniyal Vijayakumar, Pedro A Lemos,
Patrick W Serruys

Introduction

Older patients are frequently excluded from clinical studies evaluating coronary revascularization techniques. Percutaneous intervention seems to be an appealing approach for these patients, by minimizing the risk of procedure-related complications compared to more aggressive treatment modalities (e.g. surgery). Moreover, a therapeutic strategy capable of reducing the need for future revascularization is ideal, as quality of life and symptom relief might be key issues for patients of extreme age. This chapter evaluates the short- and mid-term outcomes of elderly (> 80 years) patients treated with unrestrictive utilization of sirolimus-eluting stent (SES) in the RESEARCH study.

Study population and baseline characteristics

Up to March 2003, 46 patients were treated with percutaneous coronary intervention utilizing exclusively sirolimus-eluting stents. They are analyzed in the present chapter. Baseline patient characteristics are shown. Mean age was 82±2 years (range 80–91), 57% were males, diabetes was present in 7%, hypertension in 37%, and 11% were current smokers. Previous myocardial infarction was documented in 30%, 20% had previous percutaneous interventions, and 20% previous coronary bypass surgery. Multivessel coronary disease was present in 65%. Most of the patients were admitted with an acute coronary syndrome (unstable angina in 61% and acute myocardial infarction in 9%).

Overall, 99 sirolimus-eluting stents were implanted in 90 coronary segments. The left anterior descending artery was the most commonly treated artery (58% of patients) and left main coronary artery intervention was required in 9%. Multivessel stenting was done in 37%. Also, 37% of cases received more than one stent in a single coronary artery. The average stent diameter and stent length was 2.7±0.3 mm and 17.6±8.9 mm respectively. Periprocedural glycoprotein IIb/IIIa inhibitors were used in 11%. A femoral access closure device was utilized in 40%.

Clinical outcomes

There were no major adverse events during the index hospitalization. Also, there were no in-hospital non-cardiac procedure-related complications (including major vascular complications requiring intervention or transfusion).

During the 30 day follow up there was 1 (2.2%) death, 1 (2.2%) myocardial infarction and 1 (2.2%) target vessel revascularization. One patient had sub-acute thrombotic occlusion of the stents (2.2%). After the first month, (mean follow-up period 378±69 days), there were 3 additional deaths (total death rate 8.7%), with the time between the index procedure and late (after 30 days) death ranging from 275 to 385 days. There were no late myocardial infarction (total MI rate 2.2%) and one additional patient required repeat intervention after 30 days (total re-intervention rate 4.4%). Overall, the survival rate was 91.3% and the survival free of events was 89.1% at one year (Figure 10.1).

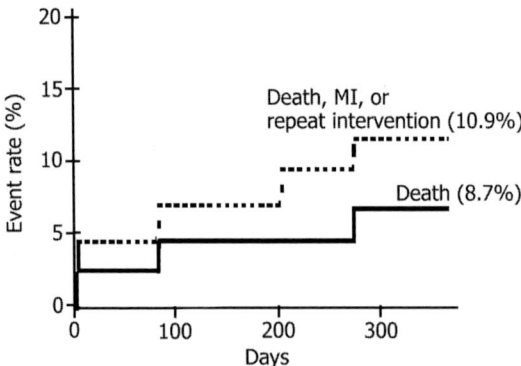

Figure 10.1 *Kaplan–Meier curves for mortality and major adverse cardiac events of elderlies treated with sirolimus-eluting stents (SES). Note that most events are due to the relatively high mortality rate of this subset, with the need for further revascularization after SES implantation accounting for only a reduced proportion of events.*

Table 10.1. Mortality and repeat revascularization rates in previous studies with elderlies treated with percutaneous intervention and in the RESEARCH.

	Mortality	Repeat intervention
De Gregorio et al.[111]	9%	28%
Kobayashi et al.[112]	13%	16%
Abizaid et al.[113]	8%	11%
Pfisterer et al.[114]	11%	10%
RESEARCH	9%	4%

Interpretation of the findings

The main findings of the present chapter are that sirolimus-eluting stent implantation in octogenarians is safe and associated with very low rates of repeat target vessel revascularization at 1 year. Older patients differ from their younger counterparts by commonly presenting with more extensive atherosclerotic disease as well as extra cardiac conditions, which may increase morbidity and mortality rates. Recent studies have previously evaluated the outcomes of elderly patients treated with invasive coronary procedures.[111–114] In the Trial of Invasive versus Medical therapy in Elderly patients (TIME) trial with elderly patients with stable angina, invasive treatment (percutaneous or surgical) reduced the risk for late re-hospitalization compared to patients randomized to medical management.[114] However, 10% of cases still needed to be re-treated during the first year follow-up. The present findings show that sirolimus-eluting stent implantation in octagenarians is associated with very low rates of repeat intervention, and highlights the promising role of the strategy for older patients (Table 10.1). Although somewhat high, the overall mortality of elderly patients in RESEARCH is in the expected range for this subset (Table 10.1). Indeed 3 out of 4 deaths were due to non-cardiac causes and occured 9 months after the index procedure.

In conclusion, sirolimus eluting stent implantation in octogenarians appears to be feasible and is associated with very low rates of subsequent repeat revascularization at one year.

III Sirolimus-Eluting Stents for Patients at Special Anatomic Groups

11. SIROLIMUS-ELUTING STENTS FOR CHRONIC TOTAL OCCLUSIONS

Angela Hoye, Kengo Tanabe, Patrick W Serruys

Introduction

Chronic total occlusions (CTO) are common, and found in approximately one third of patients with significant coronary disease who undergo angiography.[115,116] Percutaneous intervention (PCI) of CTOs accounts for 10–15% of all angioplasties; however, following successful recanalization, there is an increased rate of subsequent restenosis and re-occlusion compared to non-occlusive stenoses.[117,118] Although several randomized trials demonstrated the efficacy of stent implantation over balloon-only angioplasty; even with stents, there remains a significant rate of both restenosis (32–55%) and re-occlusion (8–12%).[119–123] This chapter examines the effectiveness of the sirolimus-eluting stents (SES) for patients with at least one *de novo* CTO treated in the RESEARCH.

Patient population and procedural characteristics

In the first 6 months of RESEARCH, 56 patients were successfully revascularized for at least one CTO with sirolimus-eluting stents and were compared with 28 patients treated with bare stents in the period before. Chronic total occlusion was defined as a complete occlusion on angiography, with no antegrade filling of the distal vessel other than via collaterals. All included patients had a native vessel occlusion estimated to be of at least 1-month duration,[123] based on either a history of sudden chest pain, a previous acute myocardial infarction in the same target vessel territory, or the time between the diagnosis made on coronary angiography and PCI. The length of the occlusion was measured by quantitative coronary angiography either by utilizing antegrade filling via collaterals, or by assessment of the retrograde collateral filling. For this, it was frequently performed a double catheterization of both the left and right coronary arteries, with simultaneous contrast injection to delineate the distance between the site of occlusion and the most proximal part of the vessel filled retrogradely.

Table 11.1. Baseline patient demographics. Reprinted from Hoye et al.[123a] With permission from the American Academy of Cardiology Foundation.

	Bare stents (n=28)	SESs (n=56)	p-value
Mean age (years)	59.8±11.1	60.2±10.0	0.9
Male sex (%)	85.7	71.4	0.2
Current smoker (%)	35.7	26.8	0.5
Diabetes mellitus (%)	7.1	14.3	0.5
Hypertension (%)	39.3	39.3	1.0
Hypercholesterolemia (%)	57.1	55.4	1.0
Previous MI (%)	46.4	55.4	0.6
Previous PCI (%)	21.4	12.5	0.3
Previous CABG (%)	0	0	–
IIb/IIIa inhibitor (%)	25.0	21.4	1.0
Multivessel disease (%)	60.7	46.3	0.3
PCI in at least one additional (non-occluded) major vessel (%)	28.6	42.6	0.2

SES: sirolimus-eluting stents, CABG: coronary artery bypass grafting, PCI: percutaneous coronary intervention

Table 11.2. Baseline procedural characteristics. Reprinted from Hoye et al.[123a] With permission from the American Academy of Cardiology Foundation.

	Bare stents (n=29)	SESs (n=56)	p value
Target vessel			0.06
LAD (%)	27.6	51.8	
LCX (%)	27.6	25.0	
RCA (%)	44.8	23.2	
Mean length of occlusion (mm), (range)	12.7 (2.4–31.8)	11.3 (4.0–32.1)	0.5
Bifurcation stenting (%)	17.9	14.3	1.0
Mean number of stents implanted	1.8	2.0	1.0
Mean stent diameter (mm)	3.03±0.56	2.75±0.26	<0.001
Mean stent length (mm)	23.3±9.3	23.9±9.2	0.7
Total stented length (mm), (range)	41.8 (18–112)	45.2 (8–117)	0.7
Post-procedure QCA data			
Reference diameter (mm)	2.37±0.50	2.35±0.46	0.9
Minimal lumen diameter (mm)	2.18±0.49	2.06±0.48	0.3
Diameter stenosis (%)	10.4	11.6	0.6

LAD=left anterior descending artery; LCX=circumflex artery, RCA=right coronary artery; QCA=quantitative coronary angiography

Table 11.3. Post-procedural and 6-month follow-up quantitative angiographic data for the sirolimus-eluting stent (n=33). Reprinted from Hoye et al.[123a] With permission from the American Academy of Cardiology Foundation.

	Proximal 5 mm	In-stent	Distal 5 mm
Post-procedure			
Mean diameter (mm)	2.82±0.66	2.58±0.55	2.10±0.64
MLD (mm)	2.43±0.51	2.04±0.45	1.75±0.53
% diameter stenosis	14.1	12.9	21.8
6 month follow-up			
MLD (mm)	2.33±0.90	1.91±0.68	1.81±0.75
% diameter stenosis	20.1	21.9	18.2
Lumen loss (mm)	0.10±0.80	0.13±0.46	−0.06±0.54

MLD=minimal luminal diameter

The baseline patient and lesion characteristics of the two groups are presented in Tables 11.1 and 11.2. One patient in the bare stent group underwent successful recanalization and stent implantation in two CTOs, thereby making a total of 29 lesions in this group. Mean length of occlusion could be determined in 45 (80.0%) of the SES group and 17 (62.1%) of the bare stent group. There was no significant difference between the groups with respect to the post-procedural quantitative angiography; however, the mean diameter of stent utilized was greater in the bare stent cohort.

Clinical and angiographic follow-up

There were no in-hospital major adverse events. During the late follow-up, there were no deaths or acute myocardial infarction in either group, with all events related to TVR. At one year, the cumulative survival-free of MACE was 96.4% in the SES group compared to 82.8% in the bare metal stent group, p<0.05. One patient in each group had a re-occlusion (1.8% SES group versus 3.6% bare stent group, p=NS).

At 6 months, 33 (58.9%) patients in the SES group underwent follow-up angiography, (none in the bare stent group). The binary restenosis rate was 9.1%: one occlusion, one stenosis at the ostium of a side branch following T-stenting, and the third at the distal outflow of the SES (Table 11.3). The patient with occlusion underwent bifurcation T-stenting following successful recanalization of a heavily calcified left anterior descending artery. At follow-up, the artery had re-occluded, and there was new akinesis of the left

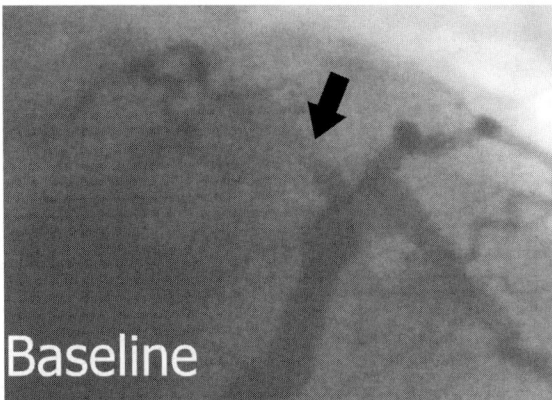

Baseline

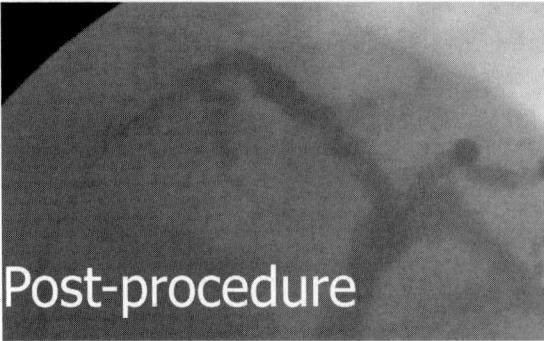

Post-procedure

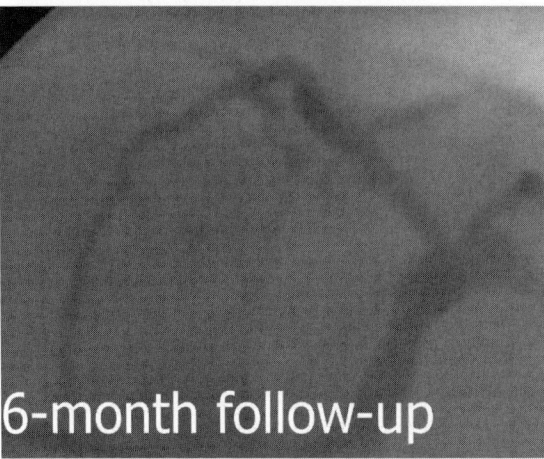

6-month follow-up

Figure 11.1 *Sirolimus-eluting stent implantation in a patient with stable angina and a chronic (>3 months) total occlusion of the left anterior descending artery (top, arrow). Two overlapping stents (2.5 × 33 mm and 2.5 × 8 mm) were successfully implanted (middle), with almost no change in the luminal dimensions at 6-month follow-up.*

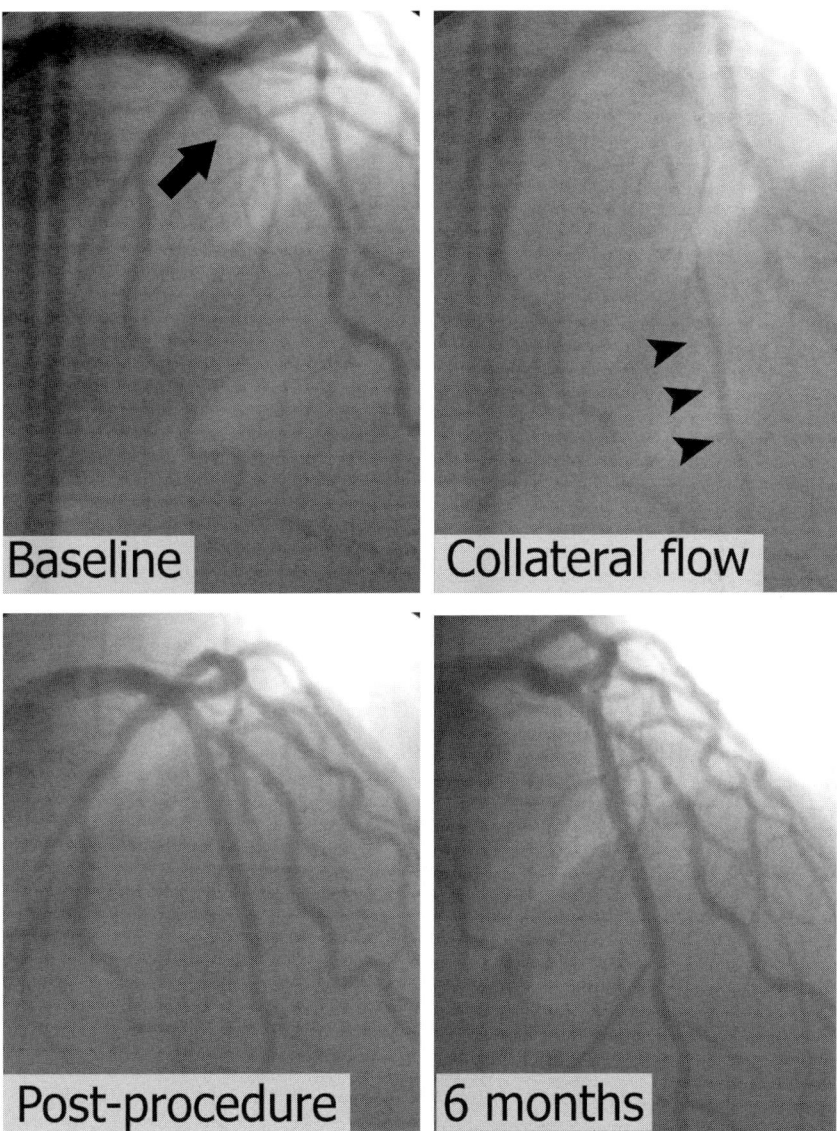

Figure 11.2 *Chronic total occlusion of the left anterior descending artery (top left, arrow), with the distal vessel filled by collateral flow (top right, arrow heads). Two sirolimus-eluting stents were implanted (both 3 × 18 mm) with good angiographic result (bottom left), which remained virtually unchanged after 6 months (bottom right).*

ventricular anterior wall. This patient with occlusion was managed with medical therapy; the other 2 patients with restenosis underwent percutaneous revascularization. Figures 11.1 and 11.2 show typical cases of a patient with CTO treated with SES.

Interpretation of the findings

Previous studies have demonstrated the importance of revascularization of CTOs, with improvement in anginal symptoms, exercise capacity, and left ventricular function.[124–126] In addition, successful recanalization reduces the subsequent need for bypass surgery, the rate of acute MI; and importantly, long-term evaluation has shown a 10-year survival advantage of 73.5% following successful PCI compared to 65.1% in those with unsuccessful PCI.[118,127]

Of the patients analyzed in this chapter, who underwent follow-up angiography, both the in-stent and proximal 5 mm segments analyzed showed an encouraging late loss of 0.13 ± 0.46 mm and 0.10 ± 0.80 mm respectively. The distal 5 mm actually showed an overall benefit, with enlargement of the vessel (late loss -0.06 ± 0.54 mm).

In addition to the angiographic data, the clinical follow-up is very encouraging with no death or myocardial infarction. Importantly, there were no significant differences in baseline demographics between the SES and bare stent groups, and all procedures were carried out in the same center by the same operators. The restenosis rate for bare stents is inversely related to the post-procedural MLD and the number of stents utilized.[128] In the present study population, although the mean diameter of stent used was significantly greater in the bare stent cohort (related to a maximum available SES diameter of 3.0 mm), with free utilization of post-dilatation, the post-procedural MLD was not significantly different between the 2 groups. All events in both groups related to TVR, and at one year, there was a significantly higher rate of survival-free of major adverse events of 96.4% in the SES group versus 82.8% in the bare stent group.

Four major randomized trials have demonstrated the efficacy of stent implantation over balloon-only angioplasty in the treatment of CTOs, reducing the 6-month restenosis rate from 68–74% to 32–55%.[119–122] Nevertheless, compared to this historical data with bare stents, the present findings suggest that the SES confers a marked further advantage with a significantly lower binary restenosis rate of 9.1% ($p<0.05$ for a comparison between the pooled previous data with bare stents[119–122] vs. the present results with SES) (Figure

84

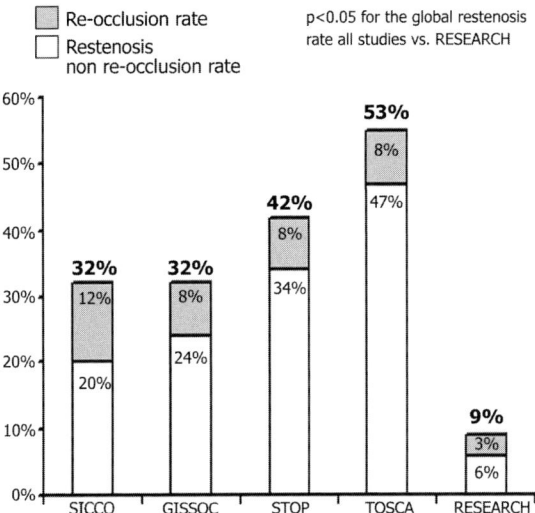

Figure 11.3 The percentage re-occlusion (gray bar), non-reoclusion restenosis (white bar), and global binary restenosis rate (top number in bold) of RESEARCH compared with published previous data from the bare stent implantation in the SICCO,[119] GISSOC,[120] STOP,[121] and TOSCA trials.[122]

11.3). In addition, we had only one patient (3.0%) with vessel re-occlusion, compared to rates of between 8–12% in the same published trials utilizing bare stents. A recent study of the clinical results of 376 patients discharged from hospital without an adverse event following successful intervention of a CTO showed, at one year follow-up, a MACE-rate of 12.2%;[129] the present findings are therefore quite remarkable, with a MACE-free survival rate of 96.4%.

In conclusion, the use of SESs in the treatment of complex patients with CTOs is associated with a reduction in the rate of major adverse cardiac events and restenosis compared to bare stents.

85

12. Sirolimus-Eluting Stents for Very Small Coronary Vessels

Pedro A Lemos, Patrick W Serruys

Introduction

The role of coronary stenting for small coronary vessels is not defined, with several randomized trials comparing stents with balloon angioplasty presenting contradictory results.[130–135] In the recent RAVEL,[18] SIRIUS,[19] E-SIRIUS,[20] and C-SIRIUS trials,[21] sirolimus-eluting stent (SES) implantation has been associated with a marked treatment effect on target lesion revascularization across the entire spectrum of vessel sizes in the included population. However, these trials were restricted to relatively large vessels (minimum stent diameter available was 2.5 mm). In a post-hoc analysis of patients enrolled in RAVEL,[136] sirolimus-eluting stents effectively inhibited neointimal proliferation independently of vessel size. Conversely, in the SIRIUS trial, patients in the lower strata of vessel diameter presented higher rates of in-stent restenosis.[19] The present chapter examines the clinical and angiographic performance of sirolimus-eluting stents dedicated to the treatment of very small vessels.

Patient population

A total of 91 consecutive patients had been treated with 2.25-mm diameter SES for 112 *de novo* lesions during the first 6 months of enrolment in RESEARCH. Among these 91 patients, 60 patients had also lesions treated with SES (2.5 mm diameter (n=109 lesions) (average stent diameter in these lesions 2.9±0.2 mm). The angiographic outcomes of lesions treated with larger SES were utilized as a reference for comparison with lesions treated with 2.25-mm SES.

Baseline clinical characteristics are shown in Table 12.1. Angiographic findings of lesions treated with 2.25-mm SES and lesions treated with larger diameter stents in other vessel segments are presented in Table 12.2. Lesions treated with 2.25-mm SESs were more frequently located at secondary

Table 12.1. Baseline and follow-up clinical characteristics of patients treated 2.25-mm diameter sirolimus-eluting stents (n=91 patients). (Reprinted from Lemos et al.[136a] With permission from Excerpta Medica, Inc.)

Men	56 (62%)
Age (years±SD)	64±12
Diabetes mellitus	24 (26%)
On insulin	9 (10%)
Systemic hypertension	51 (56%)
Current smoking	21 (23%)
Previous myocardial infarction	29 (32%)
Previous percutaneous intervention	23 (25%)
Previous coronary bypass surgery	10 (11%)
Acute coronary syndrome	34 (37%)
Multivessel coronary disease	66 (72%)
12-month follow-up	
Death	2 (2.2%)
Death + myocardial infarction	3 (3.3%)
Target lesion revascularization	5 (5.5%)
Any major adverse cardiac event	7 (7.7%)

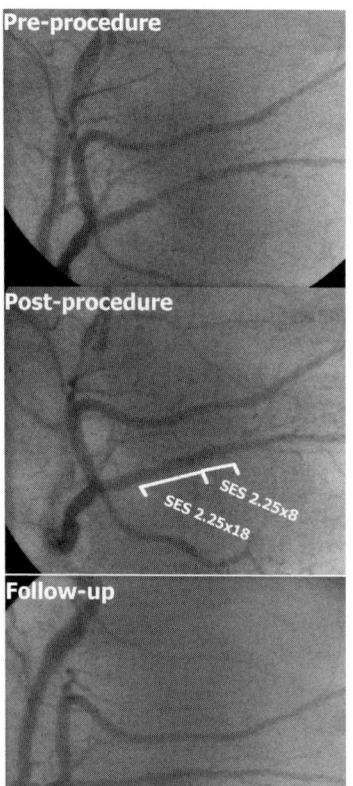

Figure 12.1 *Very small (2.25-mm) sirolimus-eluting stent (SES) implanted at the right posterior descending artery. Two SES were deployed (2.25 × 18 + 2.25 × 8) to treat a relatively long lesion. After 6 months, the patient was asymptomatic, with no evidence of restenosis at the angiographic re-study.*

Table 12.2. Angiographic characteristics of lesions treated with sirolimus-eluting stents of larger diameters and lesions treated with 2.25-mm diameter sirolimus-eluting stent. (Reprinted from Lemos et al.[136a] With permission from Excerpta Medica, Inc.)

	Larger SES (n=109)	2.25-mm SES (n=112)	p-value
Treated coronary arteries			<0.01
Left anterior descending artery	35 (32%)	18 (16%)	
Diagonal	2 (2%)	33 (30%)	
Left circumflex artery	22 (20%)	15 (13%)	
Obtuse marginal or intermedius	12 (11%)	21 (19 %)	
Right coronary artery	30 (28%)	8 (7%)	
Other branches	8 (7%)	17 (15%)	
Proximal location	34 (31%)	11 (10%)	<0.01
Ostial location	21 (19%)	47 (42%)	<0.01
Pre-procedure			
Reference diameter (mm±SD)	2.52±0.57	1.88±0.34	<0.01
Minimal luminal diameter (mm±SD)	0.82±0.53	0.57±0.37	<0.01
Diameter stenosis (%±SD)	67.8±18.5	69.4±19.1	0.5
Lesion length (mm±SD)	15.8±9.8	12.3±9.3	0.02
Post-stenting			
Minimal luminal diameter (mm±SD)	2.23±0.62	1.74±0.35	<0.01
Diameter stenosis (%±SD)	16.5±12.8	15.9±10.9	0.7
Follow-up*			
Minimal luminal diameter (mm±SD)	2.18±0.64	1.61±0.57	<0.01
Diameter stenosis (%±SD)	20.4±16.7	25.1±24.0	0.2
Late loss (mm±SD)	0.03±0.38	0.07±0.48	0.5
Binary restenosis (%)	3.9	10.7	0.1

SD=standard deviation; SES=sirolimus-eluting stent
*Refers to 62 patients (70% of eligible patients) with angiographic follow-up at 6 months (76 lesions in the larger SES group and 75 lesions in the 2.25-mm SES group)

branches, non-proximal segments, and ostial lesions, and had significantly smaller reference diameters (1.88±0.34 mm vs. 2.52±0.57 mm; p<0.01).

Clinical and angiographic follow-up

Angiographic follow-up (7.1±1.3 months) was available for 62 patients (70% of eligible patients) and 151 lesions. Late loss was similar between both lesion groups (0.07±0.48 mm for 2.25-mm SES vs. 0.03±0.38 mm for larger SES; p=0.5) (Figure 12.1). Binary restenosis was identified in 8 lesions (10.7%)

treated with 2.25-mm SESs and in 3 lesions (3.9%) treated with larger SESs (p=0.1). From the 8 restenotic lesions in 2.25-mm SESs, 3 (38%) occurred in stents implanted at the vessel ostium. Similarly, from the 3 restenotic lesions treated with larger SESs, 1 lesion (33%) was ostial. Restenosis rates for non-ostial lesions were 6.7% in the 2.25-mm SES group (n=45 lesions with angiographic follow-up) and 3.0% in the larger SES group (n=66 lesions) (p=0.4). All restenoses occurred within the stent.

Table 12.1 shows the follow-up clinical information (mean 258±92 days). There were 2 in-hospital deaths (both in patients admitted with myocardial infarction and cardiogenic shock). Non-fatal ST-elevation myocardial infarction was diagnosed in one patient (creatine phosphokinase elevation 2.8 times the upper normal limit), and occurred in the same day of the index procedure due to thrombotic occlusion of a 2.25-mm SES implanted in the distal left anterior descending artery. A distal edge dissection was seen by intravascular ultrasound examination and treated with implantation of another 2.25-mm SES overlapping the previous stent. This patient was asymptomatic after 7 months, with widely patent SESs at angiographic evaluation. There were no other cases of stent thrombosis or myocardial infarction. Target lesion revascularization was performed in another 4 patients to treat restenosis occurring after 2.25-mm SES implantation (overall target lesion revascularization rate 5.5%) and the major adverse cardiac event rate was 7.7%.

Interpretation of the findings

The present findings show that implantation of very small (2.25-mm) sirolimus-eluting stents for de novo lesions is associated with markedly low lumen loss and restenosis rates. The reduced incidence of restenosis was translated into a very low need for repeat target lesion revascularization at 12 months (5.5%).

Small vessel size has been shown to be an important independent predictor of restenosis after percutaneous intervention.[3] Currently, the best interventional approach for patients small coronary vessels is unclear, even though a number of strategies have been tested in several randomized trials.[130–135] The present chapter shows that implantation of 2.25-mm sirolimus-eluting stents strikingly inhibits neointimal proliferation in vessels with an average reference diameter of 1.88 mm, which is consistently smaller than the vessel size of all randomized studies published to date, ranging from 2.23 mm to 2.55 mm (Figure 12.2).[130–135] Although SES were implanted in very small vessels in our study, the late lumen loss (0.07 mm) was clearly smaller than

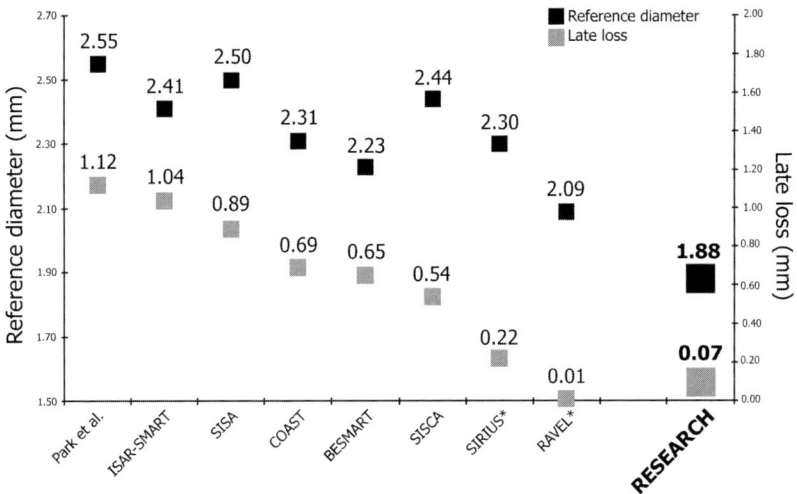

Figure 12.2 *Reference diameter and late loss in the stent arm of 6 randomized trials comparing stent implantation with balloon angioplasty for small vessels, in the SIRIUS and RAVEL trials (lowest vessel size range)*, and in the RESEARCH registry (2.25-mm sirolimus-eluting stents).*

after conventional stenting in previous series (1.12 mm to 0.54 mm).[130–135] Moreover, the late loss observed after 2.25-mm SES was similar to the late loss in previous trials with larger sirolimus-eluting stents, even when considering only vessels in the lowest tercile of vessel size were included in these studies (Figure 12.2).[19, 136]

It is worth noting that restenosis was relatively common after treatment of ostial lesions. Placement of drug-eluting stents at ostial lesions may constitute a challenging technical problem in accomplishing complete lesion scaffolding. Post-sirolimus-eluting stent restenosis is commonly associated with a discontinuity in stent coverage, which may be of particular concern for ostial (and bifurcation) lesions (see Chapter 18). Drug-eluting stents especially designed for these lesions may be needed to improve the outcomes in this setting.

In conclusion, implantation of 2.25-mm sirolimus-eluting stents in very small vessels of an unselected patient population treated in the 'real world' was associated with low rates of restenosis and a reduced incidence of target lesion revascularization.

13. SIROLIMUS-ELUTING STENTS FOR VERY LONG LESIONS

Muzaffer Degertekin, Chourmouzios A Arampatzis,
Pedro A Lemos

Introduction

Implantation of bare metal stents over a long vessel segment has long been considered to be an important risk factor for restenosis and poorer clinical outcomes.[137–143] Therefore, stent placement for diffusely diseased coronary segments is commonly avoided and is a frequent cause for deferring the percutaneous treatment. To date, randomized trials with sirolimus-eluting stents (SES) have only enrolled patients with relatively short lesion lengths. The RAVEL trial included only single lesions covered by an 18-mm long SES.[18] In the SIRIUS trial,[19] relatively longer stent placement was allowed (maximum of 2 overlapping 18-mm long SES). Similarly, the E-SIRIUS and C-SIRIUS trials[20,21] only included lesions 15–32 mm by visual assessment that could be completely covered by a maximum of two 18-mm SES. Therefore, the safety and efficacy of SES implanted over a total coronary length >36 mm has not been tested to date and is evaluated in the present chapter.

Study population

During the RESEARCH registry, SES were available at lengths of 8 mm, 18 mm, and 33 mm. In this chapter, a pre-defined study population composed of patients treated with stented segments >36 mm long is analyzed. Therefore, owing to the availability of stent lengths, all included patients had a combination of at least 2 overlapping stents in a minimum length of 41 mm (i.e. one 33-mm SES overlapping a 8-mm SES). Patients receiving SES to treat in-stent restenotic lesions were excluded from the present analysis. Also, lesions with angiographically visible gaps between stents were not included. During 6 months of enrolment, 96 consecutive patients (102 lesions) fulfilled the above criteria and are analyzed herein. The stented length was based on the cumulative length of the individual adjacent stents.

93

Clinical, procedural, and angiographic findings

Baseline and procedural characteristics of the 96 patients (102 lesions) are presented in Table 13.1. Approximately half of lesions were located in the left anterior descending coronary artery (47%) or in the right coronary artery (44%). The mean number of stents per lesion was 2.66±0.9 (range 2 to 6

Table 13.1. Demographics and procedural data (96 pts; 102 lesions). (Reprinted from Degertekin et al.[143a] With permission from Excerpta Medica, Inc.)

Age (years)	64±12
Male (%)	62
Diabetes (%)	18
Current smoking (%)	26
Hypercholesterolemia (%)	57
Hypertension (%)	45
Previous myocardial infarction (%)	32
Previous Balloon Angioplasty (%)	19
Target vessel	
Left anterior descending artery (%)	47
Left circumflex artery (%)	9
Right coronary artery (%)	44
Chronic Total Occlusion (%)	20
Direct stenting (%)	53
Primary angioplasty,(%)	8
Glycoprotein IIb/IIIa inhibitor use (%)	31
Number of stents (per lesion)	2.66±0.9 (2–6)
Stented length (per lesion), (mm [range])	61.2±21.4 (41–134)
Mean nominal stent diameter (mm, [range])	2.82±0.24

Table 13.2: Quantitative coronary angiography post-procedure and at 6 months for patients with follow-up data (n=67). (Reprinted from Degertekin et al.[143a] With permission from Excerpta Medica, Inc.)

	Proximal 5 mm	In-stent	Distal 5 mm
Post-procedure			
RD (mm)	3.17±0.55	2.68±0.51	2.45±0.51
MLD (mm)	2.76±0.54	2.17±0.47	1.94±0.53
Diameter stenosis, (%)	12	18	20
6-month follow-up			
RD (mm)	3.30±0.61	2.82±0.59	2.63±0.62
MLD (mm)	2.74±0.58	2.04±0.64	2.12±0.60
Diameter stenosis (%)	17	27	19
Late lumen loss (mm)	0.02±0.52	0.13±0.47	−0.16±0.47

MLD=Minimal lumen diameter; RD=Reference diameter

stents) and the average stented length was 61.2±21.4 mm. Angiographic success rate was 97%.

Follow-up coronary angiography was performed in 67 patients (71% of eligible cases) (Table 13.2). Binary restenosis (diameter stenosis >50%) was identified in 8 lesions (11.9%). Among the 8 lesions (8 patients) with binary restenosis, 5 occurred within the stent, 1 in the proximal and 2 in the distal 5-mm adjacent vessel segment. All post-SES restenosis were focal and less than 10 mm in length. Among these 8 patients, 4 were asymptomatic and did not undergo repeat revascularization. Figure 13.1 shows an illustrative case of a patient who received 8 overlapped stents (total length sum 104 mm) to treat a

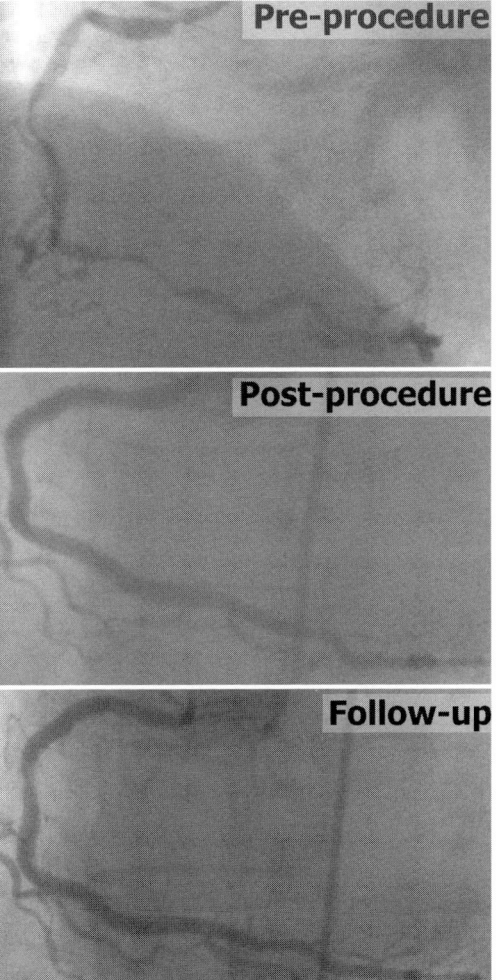

Figure 13.1 Very long length sirolimus-eluting stent (SES) implantation. The upper panel shows the right coronary artery with diffuse multifocal disease, presenting tight stenoses at its ostium, mid, and distal portions. The patient received 8 sirolimus-eluting stents to cover the entire length of the diseased vessel and a distal dissection after the implantation of the first stents, with a summed stented length of 104 mm (mid panel). The lower panel shows the late angiographic follow-up, with no evidence of neointimal proliferation.

Table 13.3. 320-day major adverse cardiac events (n=96). (Reprinted from Degertekin et al.[143a] With permission from Excerpta Medica, Inc.)

Death, n (%)	2 (2.1)
Non-fatal myocardial infarction, n (%)	1 (1.0)*
Target vessel revascularization, n (%)	6 (6.2)
percutaneous intervention	4 (4.2)
coronary artery bypass graft surgery	2 (2.1)†
Any major adverse cardiac event, n (%)	8 (8.3)

* non-Q wave myocardial infarction [CPK 567 U/l (MB: 62 U/l)].
†One of 2 patients who underwent emergency CABG for left main stem dissection died in hospital.

long lesion in the right coronary artery, which were widely patent at angiographic follow-up.

The late clinical follow-up (average of 320±67.4 days) is summarized in Table 13.3. Two patients died. One patient died during the in-hospital period after urgent bypass surgery which was due to a left main stem dissection caused by the guiding catheter. The second was admitted with post-infarction unstable and cardiogenic shock. He had 3-vessel disease, but the treatment was restricted to the culprit lesion. In total, six 2.25-mm diameter SES were implanted in the LAD/diagonal bifurcation. The patient died suddenly 43 days after the procedure. Although there is no clear evidence, in this case subacute stent thrombosis cannot be ruled out. Non-fatal myocardial infarction occurred in one patient. He developed no-reflow phenomenon after stent placement, which was resolved after intracoronary adenosine and nitroprusside infusion. At 6 months' follow-up angiography, the patient was asymptomatic and the long stented segment was patent.

In total, two patients underwent urgent bypass surgery for left main dissection. One patient died in the initial hospitalization, as mentioned above. The other was successfully treated for left main dissection, but developed cardiac tamponade after the procedure and underwent surgical pericardial drainage, during which he received a venous graft to the first obtuse marginal branch. A total of 4 patients were successfully treated with repeat PCI electively for focal restenotic lesions. The overall MACE-free survival was 91.7% at 320 days follow-up.

Interpretation of the findings

In this chapter, it is shown that the use of long length of SES implantation for *de novo* coronary lesions is associated with a low rate of major adverse cardiac

Table 13.4. RESEARCH data compared with published studies with long-length bare metal stent implantation.

	Number of patients	Stented length (mm)	Reference vessel diameter (mm)	Late lumen loss (mm)	Restenosis rate (%)
IMPULSE[140]					
Single Stent	62	32	3.04	1.18	37
Two stents	62	33	3.04	1.14	38
TULIP[141]					
IVUS Guided	73	42	2.95	1.20	23
Angiography	71	35	2.96	1.33	46
ADVANCE[139]	124	–	2.80	0.79	27
Kobayashi et al.[137]	247	52	2.95	1.41	47
RESEARCH	67	61	2.68	0.13	12

events, mainly due to a low incidence of target lesion revascularization. In particular, SES demonstrated effective suppression of neointimal hyperplasia with a late lumen loss of 0.13 mm which is substantially lower than that of major published studies with bare metal stents for long segments, ranging from 0.79 mm to 1.41 mm.[137,139–143] Accordingly, the restenosis rate observed after SES was strikingly lower than previous reports. Moreover, it is noteworthy that the average stented length in the present series from RESEARCH was at least 10 mm longer than in previous series with bare metal stents (Table 13.4 and Figure 13.2).

A longer stented segment length using bare metal stents is an independent predictor of restenosis and adverse events.[137] Long stenting is frequently associated with prolonged intra-coronary manipulation because of multiple and overlapping stent placement, which may lead to injury to the vessel wall integrity. Moreover, the greater metal density may be potentially associated with a higher degree of local vascular injury, which altogether may increase the risk of cardiac events and restenosis. Indeed, the incidence of late complications has been reported to be directly proportional to the total length of stents implanted. Previously, Schalij et al reported a 25% incidence of major adverse events for patients treated with bare metal stents in a mean stented length of 45 mm.[142] In the Additional Value of NIR Stents for Treatment of Long Coronary Lesions (ADVANCE) Study,[139] the reported MACE was 23%. The present results are reassuring, since the relatively low incidence of adverse events (8.3%) presented in our series occurred in association with a markedly long length of SES implanted (average 61 mm).

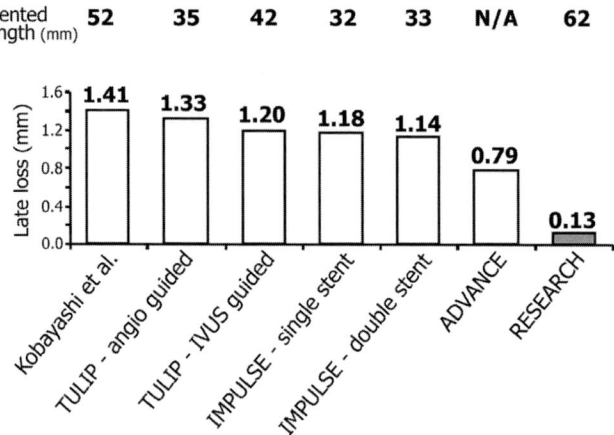

Figure 13.2 *Long lesion stenting: data from previous clinical trials* [137,139–141] *in comparison to long stenting in the RESEARCH. Note that the stented length in the RESEARCH was at least 10 mm longer than previous series with bare stents. Nevertheless, the late lumen loss after sirolimus-eluting stents in the RESEARCH was markedly lower than the historical data.*

Among 5 patients (7.4%) with in-stent restenosis, only 1 focal in-stent restenosis was seen in the overlapped stented segment. Furthermore, consistent with previous reports regarding angiographic pattern of restenosis of SES, all restenosis seen in this chapter were focal and therefore easy to treat with repeat PCI (for a detailed analysis on the pattern of post-SES restenosis, the reader is referred to Chapter 18). Since all patients with angiographically visible gaps between stents were excluded from the present analysis, incomplete lesion coverage was not identified as a possible mechanism of restenosis in any case.

There have been concerns that the risk for thrombosis might increase after implantation of long length of stent. In this chapter, no documented thrombotic stent occlusion is observed, although we cannot rule out stent thrombosis in the patient that died suddenly 43 days after the index procedure. There is no consensus for the period of clopidogrel prescription following SES implantation especially after treatment of complex lesions. Although, no late thrombotic events were diagnosed after clopidogrel discontinuation in the present series (i.e. after 6 months), additional studies are warranted to further evaluate the best antiplatelet scheme for these patients.

In conclusion, sirolimus eluting stent implantation appears to be a safe and effective treatment for *de novo* coronary lesions requiring multiple stent placement over a very long vessel segment.

14. SIROLIMUS-ELUTING STENTS FOR BIFURCATION LESIONS

Kengo Tanabe, Angela Hoye, Patrick W Serruys

Introduction

Percutaneous coronary intervention of bifurcation lesions is associated with lower procedural success rates,[144] and an increased subsequent rate of major adverse cardiac events (MACE) and restenosis. Various techniques and strategies have been applied in an attempt to improve outcomes including kissing balloon dilatation, and the use of stent implantation in both branches.[145] The use of adjunctive atherectomy was found to be not advantageous in the Coronary Angioplasty Versus Excisional Atherectomy (CAVEAT) I trial.[146] Although there was an improved initial angiographic result with less residual stenosis, this was at the expense of a higher rate of side branch occlusion and acute myocardial infarction. In the long-term, results of angioplasty in bifurcations have been hampered by problems of restenosis particularly following stent implantation within the side branch.[147,148] This chapter examines the safety and efficacy of sirolimus-eluting stents (SES) for patients with *de novo* bifurcation lesions enrolled in the RESEARCH registry.

Patient population and bifurcation techniques

The present chapter evaluates a total of 58 patients with 65 *de novo* bifurcation lesions treated with SES implantation in both the main and side branches during the first 6 months of RESEARCH. The final choice of the bifurcation stenting strategy and the use of kissing balloon dilatation were left to the operators' discretion. One of 4 methods of stenting was used: T-stenting, culotte stenting, kissing stents, or the 'crush' technique. T- and culotte stenting have been previously described.[148,149] Kissing stents involved simultaneous implantation of the stents within both branches, with the proximal edges alongside each other thereby bringing forward the point of divergence. The 'crush' technique involves positioning both stents with the proximal part of the side branch stent lying well within the main vessel, while ensuring that the edge of the stent in the main vessel is more proximal than the side branch stent. The side branch stent is deployed first, and the balloon and wire carefully withdrawn. The main vessel stent is then deployed thereby crushing the proximal part of the side branch stent.[150]

Clinical and angiographic findings

Baseline patient characteristics are summarized in Table 14.1. The lesion characteristics and stenting technique utilized are documented in Table 14.2. At

Table 14.1. Baseline Clinical Characteristics (n=58)

Age (years)	63 ± 10
Men	42 (72%)
Hypertension	26 (45%)
Hypercholesterolemia	35 (60%)
Diabetes mellitus	16 (28%)
Current smoker	16 (28%)
Previous myocardial infarction	22 (38%)
Previous coronary angioplasty	5 (9%)
Previous coronary artery bypass surgery	3 (5%)
Number of coronary arteries significantly narrowed	
1	15 (26%)
2	28 (48%)
3	15 (26%)
Acute coronary syndrome	18 (31%)

Values are presented as the numbers (relative percentages) or mean value ± SD.

Table 14.2. Procedural and Lesion Characteristics (n = 65 lesions)

Coronary artery treated with bifurcation stenting	
Left anterior descending/diagonal	39 (60%)
Left circumflex/obtuse marginal	16 (25%)
Right coronary/posterior descending	4 (6%)
Left main stem – left anterior descending/circumflex	6 (9%)
Stenting technique	
T-stenting	41 (63%)
Culotte stenting	5 (8%)
Kissing stenting	2 (3%)
Crush stenting	17 (26%)
Kissing balloon dilatation after stenting	20 (31%)
Glycoprotein IIb/IIIa inhibitor use	20 (31%)

Values are presented as the numbers (relative percentages).

6 months, the survival-free of MACE was 89.7%. One patient died following bifurcation stent implantation of the left main stem for an acute myocardial infarction. He was admitted in cardiogenic shock, and despite the use of abciximab and intra-aortic balloon pump support, died shortly after the procedure owing to left ventricular failure. There were no episodes of acute or subacute stent thrombosis, and no patient had a myocardial infarction. Target lesion revascularization was undertaken in 5 patients (8.6%) as outlined below.

Of 65 lesions, 6-month angiographic follow-up was performed in 44 lesions. The binary restenosis rate was 22.7% (10 of 44 lesions). QCA data are presented in Table 14.3. Angiographic restenosis occurred in 4 lesions within the main branch (1 in the proximal segment; 3 in the in-stent segment), yielding a restenosis rate of 9.1%. Angiographic restenosis occurred in 6 of the side branches, all within the in-stent segment. Of these 6 restenoses, 5 occurred at the ostium of side branch following the use of T-stenting (Figure 14.1). All 4 patients with a restenosis within the main vessel, and 1 patient with a restenosis at the ostium of a side branch, underwent percutaneous target lesion revascularization with new drug-eluting stent implantation. Directional coronary atherectomy was additionally used in 1 patient. The

Table 14.3. Quantitative Coronary Angiography

	Proximal	In-stent	Distal
Main branch (n = 44)			
Reference diameter (mm)	N/A	2.64	N/A
Minimal lumen diameter (mm)			
Pre-procedure	N/A	0.64	N/A
Post-procedure	2.39	2.19	1.86
6-month follow-up	2.26	2.07	1.85
Diameter stenosis at 6-month (%)	28.3	22.9	25.4
Late lumen loss (mm)	0.12	0.12	0.01
Restenosis rate (%)	2.3	6.8	0
Side branch (n =44)			
Reference diameter (mm)	–	1.99	N/A
Minimal lumen diameter (mm)	–		
Pre-procedure	–	0.61	N/A
Post-procedure	–	1.80	1.57
6-month follow-up	–	1.49	1.47
Diameter stenosis at 6-month (%)	–	31.0	21.9
Late lumen loss (mm)	–	0.31	0.09
Restenosis rate (%)	–	13.6	0

Values are presented as mean values or relative percentages

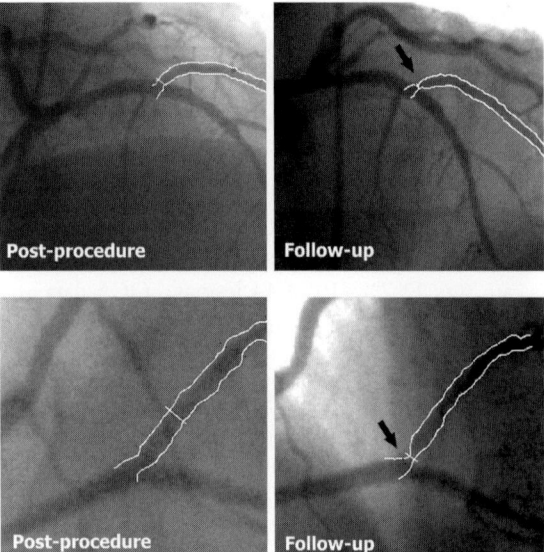

Figure 14.1 *Ostial restenosis after sirolimus-eluting stent (SES) implantation in bifurcation lesions. The figure shows the cases of two patients receiving SESs in the main vessel and in ostium of a side branch, with good acute angiographic result (left panels). At follow-up, there was no visible neointimal proliferation in the main vessels, while both side branches presented tight re-narrowing at their ostia (right panels, arrow).*

remaining 5 patients, all with ostial side branch restenosis, were asymptomatic and treated with medical therapy alone.

Interpretation of the findings

The major findings of this chapter are:

(1) SES implantation in both the main and side branches is feasible and associated with a low procedural complication rate, and no episodes of stent thrombosis.
(2) The target lesion revascularization rate of 8.6% is seemingly diminished as compared to historical controls.
(3) Angiographic restenosis rates of the main and side branches are 9.1% and 13.6%, with an overall restenosis rate of 22.7%.
(4) Five of the 6 restenoses occurring in the side branch were located at the ostium following T-stenting technique.

These findings are in line with a recent study that randomized 86 bifurcation lesions to double SES implantation of the main vessel+side branch versus SES of the main vessel with provisional stenting of the side branch.[151] The restenosis rates were not different between patients actually receiving double-stenting (28.0%) and the patients treated with provisional side branch stenting (18.7%). Most commonly, the restenosis occurred at the ostium of the side branch and were of short length (focal).

When treating bifurcation lesions with sirolimus-eluting stents with the culotte, kissing, or crush stenting techniques, there are some overlapping stent struts. At these sites, higher concentration of sirolimus may induce endothelial

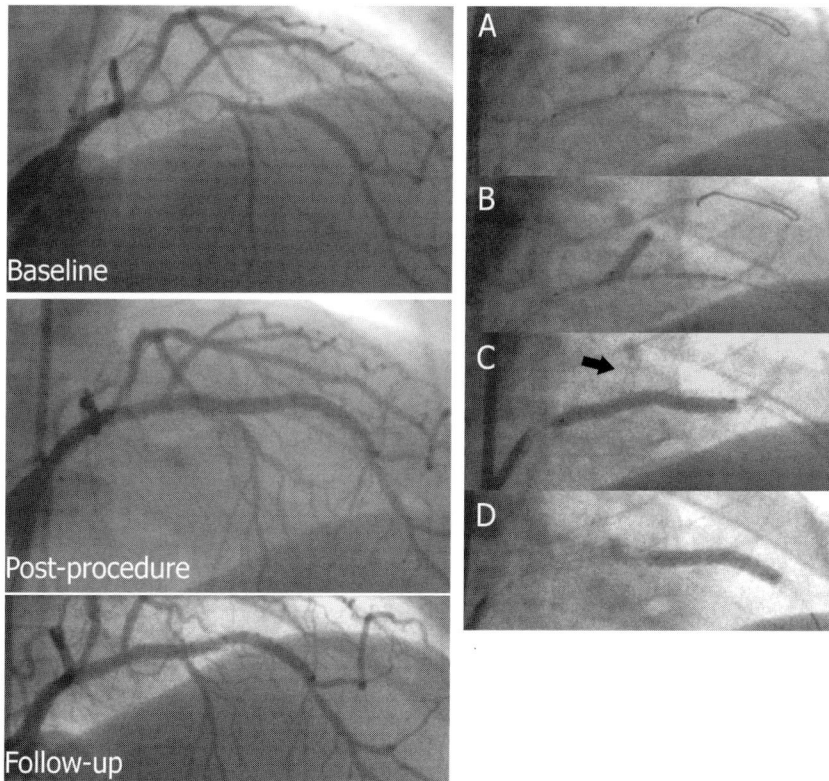

Figure 14.2 *Long stenotic segment of the left anterior descending (LAD) artery involving the ostium of the first diagonal branch (left top). Two sirolimus-eluting stents were implanted with a 'T-stenting' technique over the bifurcation site (right panels A, B, and C). Panel C shows the deployment of the stent in the LAD (the silhouette of the stent implanted in the diagonal branch is evident [black arrow]). An additional stent was implanted more distally in the LAD to cover the entire diseased segment (right panel D), and a good final angiographic result was achieved (left mid). After 6 months, the patient was asymptomatic, and the stents was widely patent (left bottom).*

103

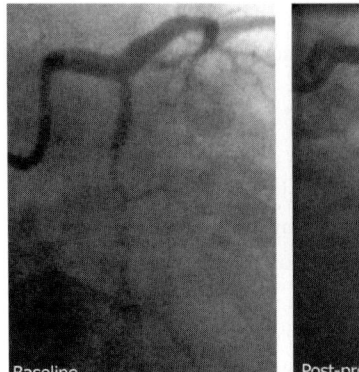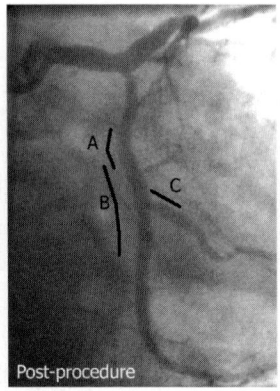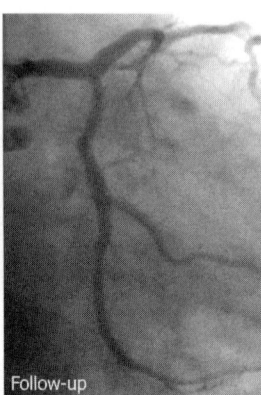

Baseline   Post-procedure   Follow-up

Figure 14.3 *Chronic total occlusion of the left circumflex artery (left panel). The bifurcation left circumflex/obtuse marginal was treated with implantation of two overlapping sirolimus-eluting stents in the circumflex (mid panel, A and B) and one stent in the marginal branch (mid panel, C) with a 'T-stenting' technique. At late follow-up, all stents were open with no angiographic evidence of neointimal proliferation.*

function impairment and thus may be, in theory, associated with an increased risk of stent thrombosis. Although these stenting techniques were applied in 37% of the lesions treated, no stent thrombosis was reported during the follow-up period, implying that sirolimus has a wide safety margin.

Several strategies have been advocated to treat bifurcation lesions with PCI, such as deployment of stents in both vessels, stenting in one branch with balloon angioplasty in the other, and mechanical debulking. The published reports regarding the subsequent need for target lesion revascularization utilizing bare stents range from 17% to 53%,[148,152,153] thus the rate of 8.6% in the present series is therefore very favorable (Figures 14.2, 14.3, and 14.4). In addition, the rate observed in the current study may underestimate the true beneficial treatment effect of SES as explained below.

Five of the 6 restenoses in the side branch occurred at the ostium following T-stenting. When we apply T-stenting, stent positioning must be extremely accurate to ensure complete coverage of the side branch ostium. This is particularly difficult/impossible to achieve when the angle between the 2 branches is <90°. Restenosis at this site may therefore be mainly a reflection of incomplete coverage. The restenosis rate in the side branch following T-stenting was 16.7% (5 of 30 lesions), while that following the other stent techniques was 7.1% (1 of 14 lesions). These results suggest that it seems wise to ensure the complete coverage of the ostium with SES using stenting

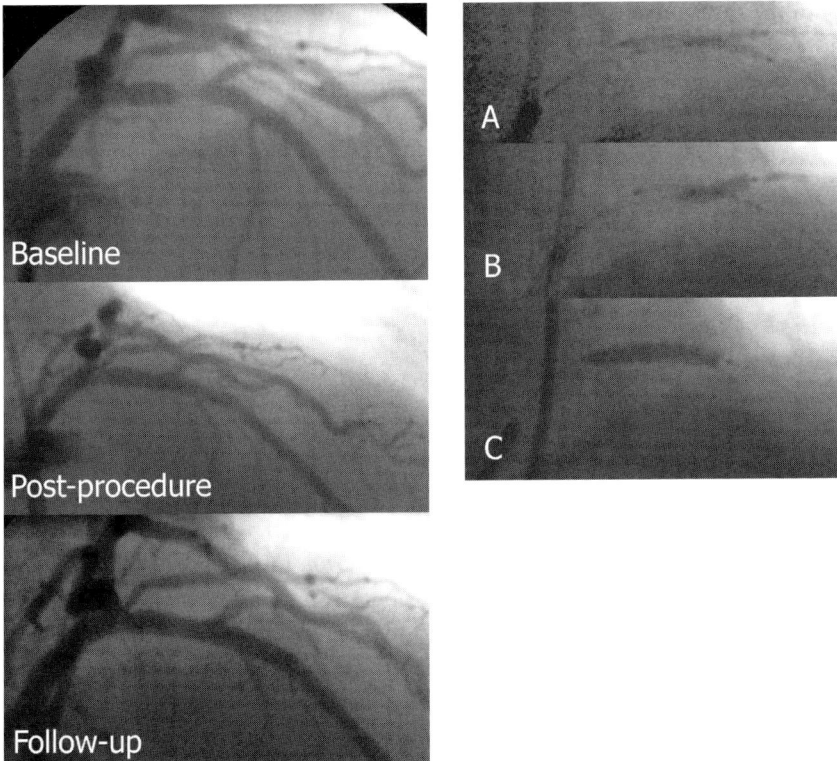

Figure 14.4 Sirolimus-eluting stent implantation at the left anterior descending (LAD)/diagonal bifurcation utilizing the 'crush' technique. Note that both stents are positioned simultaneously at the bifurcation site, with the stent at the diagonal protruding towards the lumen of the left anterior descending artery (right panel A). The stent in the diagonal was deployed first (right panel B), while the stent in the LAD was kept steady. The LAD stent is then deployed, 'crushing' the stent just deployed in the diagonal (with its proximal portion partially at the LAD) (right panel C). The acute final angiographic result was maintained virtually unchanged at 6 months.

techniques other than T-stenting. The 'crush' technique is technically easier and quicker to do than a culotte, but further data with longer follow-up from a larger population is needed to fully determine the efficacy of these techniques.

In conclusion, the percutaneous treatment of coronary bifurcation stenoses is hampered by an increased rate of subsequent restenosis. The present chapter reports on the outcomes of a consecutive series of unselected patients with *de novo* bifurcation stenoses, treated with sirolimus-eluting stent implantation in

16. SIROLIMUS-ELUTING STENTS FOR IN-STENT RESTENOSIS

Francesco Saia, Patrick W Serruys

Introduction

Treatment of in-stent restenosis is frequently a challenging clinical problem, with recurrent restenosis being reported in up to 80% in the most complex cases.[4] Currently, vascular brachytherapy is the only strategy proven to be more effective for the treatment of in-stent restenosis than other conventional approaches.[167–171] However, post-brachytherapy recurrent restenosis has been reported to occur in 17% to 32% of patients at 1 year.[167–171] Moreover, despite the relative improvement in outcomes, brachytherapy has not been extensively adopted as routine therapy in many centers, mostly because of logistic and technical limitations.

Promising results have been recently reported with sirolimus-eluting stents (SES) for the treatment of in-stent restenosis.[31,32] A relatively low incidence of repeat restenosis has been shown after drug-eluting stent implantation in these preliminary series of cases. However, the clinical efficacy of SES has not been compared to conventional percutaneous techniques or to the 'gold standard' vascular brachytherapy. Also, the impact of SES implantation for patients after 'failed' brachytherapy is uncertain.

The present chapter describes the outcomes of patients with in-stent restenosis treated with sirolimus-eluting stents in comparison to a series of patients treated with vascular brachytherapy. In an additional analysis, the impact of SES implantation for patients with previous failed brachytherapy is detailed separately.

Study population

In the first six months enrolment of RESEARCH, 44 consecutive patients with in-stent restenosis and no previous brachytherapy at the same site were treated with SES implantation. The clinical outcomes of these patients were compared to a group composed of 43 patients treated with vascular brachytherapy in the months immediately prior. Angiographic follow-up re-study was obtained from patients treated with SES only.

Separately from the analysis above, a group of 18 patients with previous failed brachytherapy treated with SES is also described in this chapter. These patients were treated during separate time periods. A first cohort was treated between March 2001 and June 2001, as part of a pilot study on SESs for treatment of in-stent restenosis. The latter cohort comprises patients treated during RESEARCH.

Table 16.1. Baseline clinical characteristics and demographics of patients without previous brachytherapy treated with SES or VBT. Catheterization and Cardiovascular Interventions. © 2004

	VBT (n. 43)	SES (n. 44)	p value
Age, y	61±10	63±13	ns
Males, n (%)	31 (73)	32 (73)	ns
Diabetes Mellitus, n (%)	11 (26)	11 (25)	ns
Hypertension, n (%)	13 (30)	21 (48)	ns
Hypercholesterolemia, n (%)	26 (60)	30 (68)	ns
Previous MI, n (%)	20 (47)	23 (52)	ns
Previous CABG, n (%)	9 (21)	10 (23)	ns
Multivessel disease, n (%)	20 (47)	22 (50)	ns
Clinical presentation, n (%)			ns
Stable Angina	34 (79)	32 (73)	
ACS	9 (21)	12 (27)	
Number of ISR lesions treated	44	53	-
ISR lesions treated per patient	1.0±0.2	1.2±0.5	0.02
Target Vessel, n (%)			ns
LAD	16 (36)	26 (49)	
LCX	9 (20)	6 (11)	
RCA	15 (34)	14 (26)	
LM	1 (2)	1 (2)	
Bypass grafts	3 (7)	6 (11)	
Mehran classification, n (%)			
Type I	10 (23)	22 (42)	0.05
Type II	19 (43)	11 (21)	0.02
Type III	10 (23)	14 (26)	ns
Type IV	5 (11)	6 (11)	ns
Multivessel procedure, n (%)	9 (21)	11 (25)	ns
Procedural success*, n (%)	42 (98)	43 (98)	ns
IIb/IIIa inhibitors, n (%)	14 (33)	4 (9)	0.007
Clopidogrel prescription, mo	7.5±5.5	5.9±2.6	0.005

ACS=Acute Coronary syndromes; CABG=Coronary Artery Bypass Graft; LAD=left anterior descending artery; LCX=left circumflex artery; MI=Myocardial Infarction; RCA=right coronary artery; LM=left main stem; TL=Target Lesion
*as judged by the operator, in the absence of in-hospital complications.

Comparison between SES versus brachytherapy for in-stent restenosis without previous brachytherapy

Baseline and procedural characteristics

The baseline characteristics of patients treated with SES or vascular brachytherapy were similar (Table 16.1). Specifically, no difference was observed in the incidence of diabetes (26% vascular brachytherapy vs. 25% SES; p=0.1), previous myocardial infarction (47% vascular brachytherapy vs. 52% SES; p=0.6), previous coronary artery bypass graft (CABG) surgery (21% vascular brachytherapy vs. 23% SES; p=0.8), or multivessel disease (47% vascular brachytherapy vs. 50% SES; p=0.7). The majority of the patients in both groups had stable angina at hospital admission (79% vascular brachytherapy vs. 73% SES; p=0.5). Almost all patients in the VBT group had single-lesion brachytherapy, except by one patient with 2 lesions treated. In the SES group, 53 in-stent restenosis lesions were treated (1.2±0.5 lesion per patient). In the SES group there were more lesions classified as Mehran type I (23% vascular brachytherapy vs. 42% SES; p=0.05), while type II was more common in the vascular brachytherapy group (43% vascular brachytherapy vs. 21% SES; p=0.02). However, both treatment groups had similar numbers of lesions with non-complex (Mehran Type I/II: 66% vascular brachytherapy vs. 63% SES) or complex (Mehran Type III/IV: 34% vascular brachytherapy vs. 37% SES; p=0.7 for all) morphologies. Quantitative coronary analysis did not show significant differences in baseline lesions' characteristics between the two groups (Table 16.2). Average lesion length was 15.7±10.4 mm in the vascular

Table 16.2. Quantitative coronary analysis at baseline of patients without previous brachytherapy treated with SES or VBT. Catheterization and Cardiovascular Interventions. © 2004

	VBT (n. 44)	SES (n. 53)	p value
Pre-procedure			
Reference diameter, mm	2.44±0.45	2.64±0.56	ns
MLD, mm	0.74±0.52	0.90±0.55	ns
Diameter stenosis, %	69±20	66±19	ns
Lesion length, mm	15.7±10.4	17.5±12.1	ns
Post-procedure			
Reference diameter, mm	2.61±0.51	2.73±0.54	ns
MLD, mm	1.84±0.41	2.33±0.59	0.0008
Diameter stenosis, %	28±12	16±15	0.004

MLD = Minimal Lumen Diameter

brachytherapy group and 17.5±12.1 mm in the SES group (p=0.4). As expected, post-procedure minimal lumen diameter was bigger (1.84±0.41 mm vascular brachytherapy vs. 2.33±0.59 mm SES; p=0.0008) and diameter stenosis smaller (28±12% vascular brachytherapy vs. 16±15% SES; p=0.004) in the SES group.

In the VBT group average irradiated length was 48±12 mm, and average radiation dose administered was 23±2 Gy. A new stent was implanted in 27% of the VBT patients. In the SES group each patient received on average 2.0±1.4 stents, with a mean stent length of 28±20 mm per lesion. In the VBT group periprocedural glycoprotein IIb/IIIa inhibitors utilization was more common (33% vs. 9%; p=0.007), and clopidogrel prescription longer (7.5±5.5 months vs. 5.9±2.6 months; p=0.005).

Clinical outcomes

During nine months of follow-up, 3 patients (7%) died in the vascular brachytherapy group and 0 in the SES group (p=0.08 by log rank) (Table 16.3). They were all thought to be cardiac deaths: one patient with previous coronary bypass operation developed severe hypotension after balloon angioplasty and irradiation of the right coronary artery and died 2 days after the procedure; two patients had a sudden death 3 months after treatment of a lesion in the proximal left anterior descending while still on combined antiplatelet treatment (one of them had a new stent implanted during the brachytherapy procedure). Subacute stent thrombosis could not be ruled out in these last 2 cases. A definite diagnosis of acute MI was made in 1 patient in each group. Target lesion revascularization (TLR) was performed in 5 patients (11.6%) in the vascular brachytherapy group, and 7 patients (16.3%) in the

Table 16.3. Nine-month clinical outcome of patients without previous brachytherapy treated with SES or VBT. Catheterization and Cardiovascular Interventions. © 2004

	VBT (n. 43)	SES (n. 44)
All MACE, %	20.9	18.6
Death, %	7.0	0
Myocardial infarction, %	2.3	2.3
Target Lesion Revascularization, %	11.6	16.3
Target Vessel Revascularization, %	4.7	4.7
Coronary bypass graft, %	7.0	2.3
Percutaneous coronary intervention, %	9.3	18.6
MACE=Major Adverse Cardiovascular Events		

SES group (p=NS). In the vascular brachytherapy group these recurrent restenosis were treated with 2 CABG operations, 1 balloon angioplasty, 1 stent implantation, and 1 sirolimus-eluting stent implantation. In the SES group 1 patient underwent urgent surgery for vessel dissection and acute occlusion during treatment of a lesion in the proximal left circumflex artery, and the remaining 6 TLRs were accomplished percutaneously (3 with additional SES implantation, 3 with taxol-eluting stent implantation). Overall, the global rate of major adverse cardiac events at 9 months was similar in both groups (20.9% vascular brachytherapy vs. 18.5% SES; p=0.8).

Angiographic outcomes

Angiographic follow-up was obtained from patients treated with SES only. In total, 33 patients (41 lesions) treated with SES for in-stent restenosis without previous brachytherapy were re-studied (77% of patients and 79% of lesions with successful index procedure). The pre-procedure, post-procedure and follow-up quantitative angiographic data of this subset are shown in Table 16.4. Representative sequences of angiograms are shown in Figures 16.1 and 16.2. Mean reference diameter was 2.64±0.56 mm and mean lesion length was 17.5±12.1 mm. Late loss was 0.17±0.76 mm. Overall, post-SES binary restenosis was observed in 14.6% of the lesions. Table 16.5 shows the frequency of post-SES restenosis for some subgroups. No restenosis was observed in Mehran class I lesions; class II, III and IV lesions had post-SES restenosis in 22%, 25% and 20%, respectively (p=NS). In 5 out of 6 cases

Table 16.4. Quantitative angiographic analysis at baseline, post-procedure and follow-up of patients without previous brachytherapy treated with SES*.

	Pre-procedure	Post-procedure	Follow-up
Reference diameter, mm	2.64±0.56	2.73±0.54	2.83±0.50
Minimum lumen diameter, mm	0.90±0.55	2.33±0.59	2.20±0.81
Diameter stenosis, %	66±19	16±15	23±25
Lesion length, mm	17.5±12.1	–	–
Acute gain, mm	–	1.42±0.70	-
Late loss, mm	–	–	0.17±0.76
Late loss excluding occlusions, mm	–	–	0.11±0.67
Post-SES restenosis†, %			14.6

SES=sirolimus-eluting stent
*related to 41 lesions with angiographic follow-up
†including one total re-occlusion

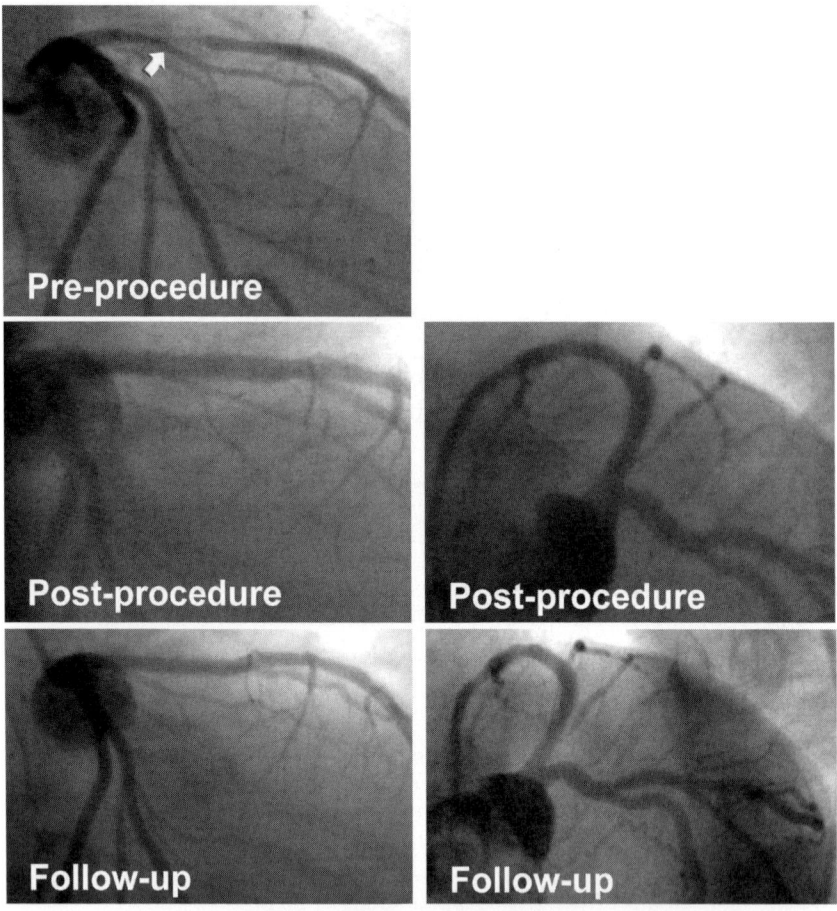

Figure 16.1 In-stent restenosis at the proximal left anterior descending artery (arrow, upper panel) of a stent implanted 6 months before. The patient was admitted with moderate stable angina and was treated with direct stent implantation of a 3.0 × 23 sirolimus-eluting stent (post-dilatation with a 3.5-mm balloon), with good final angiographic result (mid panel). After 6 months, the patient was asymptomatic and angiographic follow-up revealed no evidence of neointimal proliferation at the treated site.

with post-SES restenosis the restenosis was focal or multifocal. For patients with post-SES restenosis, the average lesion length decreased from 31.7±15.3 mm at baseline to 10.0±4.8 mm at follow-up (p=0.01). One patient presented post-SES with silent total occlusion. Post-SES restenotic lesions were located within the SES in 5 lesions and at the proximal edge in

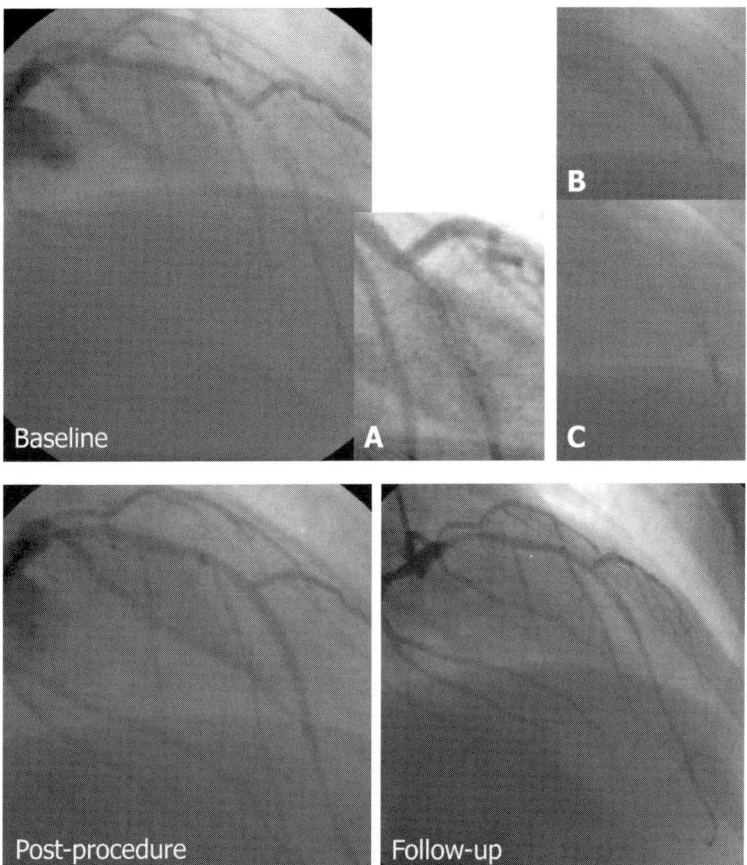

Figure 16.2 *Long in-stent restenosis (left top) of a stent implanted 6 months before at the left anterior descending artery (the old stent struts are visible in panel A). Two overlapping sirolimus-eluting stents (2.75 × 33 mm [panel B] and 2.5 × 8 mm [panel C]) were successfully implanted (left bottom). At 6-month angiographic follow-up, both stents were open without recurrent restenosis.*

the remaining 1. In two patients, post-SES restenosis occurred in an uncovered region injured during the procedure (gap between two SES implanted to treat two separate lesions in one patient and stent discontinuity by ultrasound examination due to possible stent fracture in another case). Marked SES undersizing (stent diameter 2.7 mm; vessel diameter 5.7 mm) was found in another patient with post-SES restenosis.

The patients that developed post-SES restenosis had baseline clinical characteristics similar to the others. However, the lesions who developed

119

Table 16.5. Binary post-SES restenosis in subgroups of patients without previous brachytherapy treated with SES*

	Post-SES restenosis
Total population (n=41)	14.6%
Diabetics (n=8)	25.0%
Small vessel size (n=20) †	10.0%
Vein grafts (n=5)	20.0%
Lesion length > 20 mm (n=14)	28.6%
Bifurcating stents‡ (n=7)	14.3%
Mehran class 2	
Type I (n=15)	0
Type II (n=9)	22.2%
Type III (n=12)	25.0%
Type IV (n=5)	20.0%

Numbers in parenthesis are related to lesions with follow-up
* related to 41 lesions with angiographic follow-up
† pre-procedure reference diameter ≤2.5 mm
‡ related only to the in-stent restenosis lesions; in these series, there was no case of restenosis in the side-branches treated for de novo lesions.

binary restenosis were considerably longer (29.1±15.0 mm vs. 16.1±11.0 mm, p=0.01), were treated with more stents (2.2±0.7 vs. 1.5±0.7, p=0.04), and the stented segment was longer (average stent length per lesion: 49.0±30.0 mm vs. 25.5±16.3 mm, p<0.01) compared to lesions who presented less than 50% diameter stenosis at follow-up.

Sirolimus-eluting stents for failed brachytherapy

Baseline and procedural characteristics

Baseline characteristics of the 18 patients (18 lesions) treated with SES for failed vascular brachytherapy are listed in Table 16.6. Nine patients (50%) had had more than 2 previous episodes of restenosis. Median time from the preceding percutaneous reintervention was 678 days (range 1,111 to 1,678 days). Remarkably, 61% of cases presented with a proliferative pattern of restenosis, 44% of whom had a totally occluded target vessel. The mean length of SES implanted was 36.9±30 mm and the average stent diameter was 2.8±0.3 mm.

120

Table 16.6. Baseline and procedural characteristics and demographics of patients with failed brachytherapy SES.

Patients	18
Age, years	63±11
Men	78%
Diabetes mellitus	28%
Acute coronary syndromes	44%
Multivessel coronary disease	78%
Previous myocardial infarction	67%
Previous coronary bypass	44%
Time from last target lesion revascularization, (d)	111–1678 (678)
Time from brachytherapy, (d)	111–1968 (755)
> 2 episodes of in-stent restenosis	50%
Restenosis Mehran class	
Focal	22%
Diffuse	17%
Proliferative	17%
Total occlusion	44%

Values are mean±SD, range (median), or number of patients (%)

Clinical and angiographic outcomes

There were no in-hospital complications. At 12 months, 5 patients (28%) had at least one major adverse cardiac event. Two patients died (11%), 3 patients had target lesion revascularization (17%), and 3 other patients (17%) had a repeat procedure in the target vessel but outside the index lesion. Therefore, in total, 6 patients (34%) had a re-intervention in the target vessel treated at the index procedure. There were no acute, subacute, or late thromboses. Late angiographic follow-up data were obtained from 89% of patients and are shown in Table 16.7. The binary restenosis rate was 37.5% and the average late luminal loss was 0.71 mm. Two patients had a totally occluded target vessel.

Interpretation of the findings

Vascular brachytherapy has been rightly considered the gold-standard treatment for in-stent restenosis, at the least for more complex cases, after several randomized trials have shown its superiority over other conventional approaches.[167–170,172] Despite these favorable results, brachytherapy has not been widely utilized, being still currently restricted, at least in Europe, to a limited

121

Table 16.7. Quantitative angiographic analysis at baseline, post-procedure and follow-up of patients with failed brachytherapy SES*.

	Pre-procedure	Post-procedure	Follow-up
Reference diameter, mm	2.82±0.52	2.81±0.46	2.89±0.40
Minimum lumen diameter, mm	0.61±0.75	2.39±0.48	1.75±1.13
Diameter stenosis, %	79±26	14±11	40±36
Lesion length, mm	23.4±20.2	–	–
Acute gain, mm	–	1.78±0.63	-
Late loss†, mm	–	–	0.71±1.09
Post-SES restenosis†, %			37.5

SES=sirolimus-eluting stent
*related to 89% of lesions with angiographic follow-up
†including 2 total re-occlusions

number of centers. Complex logistic and technical requirements, as well as lack of reimbursement in some countries, have limited a more generalized utilization of brachytherapy. Furthermore, the identification of possible shortcomings such as geographical miss[173] and delayed re-endothelialization, which is associated with an increased risk of subacute thrombosis especially when a new stent is implanted,[174] have made mandatory specific training for the operators involved in brachytherapy procedures.

In this chapter, treatment of in-stent restenosis with sirolimus-eluting stents was associated with similar clinical results at 9 months compared to vascular brachytherapy. It is important to recognize that, differently from brachytherapy, routine utilization of sirolimus-eluting stent implantation does not deviate from the standard practice with conventional bare stents. Indeed, no additional requirements are needed to readily apply this new therapy at any catheterization laboratory.

In the evaluation of the present results that compare SES vs. vascular brachytherapy for patients with in-stent restenosis without previous brachytherapy, two additional pieces of information should be taken into account. Although not statistically significant, a slightly higher rate of TLR was observed in the SES group compared to brachytherapy treatment. However, in the former group, routine angiographic follow-up was scheduled by protocol, and performed in 77% of the patients, while only a minority of patients in the vascular brachytherapy group underwent elective angiography (30%). It has been previously shown that angiographic follow-up has a negative impact on clinical outcome which is due to more repeat revascularization procedures ('oculo-stenotic reflex').[28] Furthermore, a late 'catch-up' phenomenon (continuous increasing of angiographic late-loss after 6 months) has been reported for vascular brachytherapy,[175,176] while data regarding SES for *de novo*[16] lesions suggest that the early results are predictive of the long-term findings. On the other hand, although not statistically significant, an increased mortality was observed in the brachytherapy group (vascular brachytherapy: 7%; SES: 0%; p=0.08), suggesting once again the possibility of serious adverse events related to the prolonged endothelial damage after vessel irradiation.

The outcomes of patients with in-stent restenosis after repeat treatment have been reported to be closely related to the baseline lesion morphology.[4] A progressive increase in risk profile occurs from lesions with a focal pattern to lesions with a more diffuse appearance and total occlusions.[4] Accordingly, in our series, SES was associated with a remarkably low incidence of recurrent restenosis in focal lesions (without previous brachytherapy). Indeed, all cases of repeat restenosis occurred in patients with more complex baseline characteristics. However, no clear differences in the rates of repeat restenosis were noted among higher risk categories (i.e. Mehran classes II, III, and IV), in whom the rates of repeat restenosis have been reported to be 35%, 50% and 85%, respectively, with conventional therapy. Thus, it is possible that SES implantation may reduce the prognostic value of the lesion pattern of in-stent restenoses for non-focal in-stent restenosis, although the limited number of our observations does not allow a definitive conclusion. Conversely, the present data suggest that lesion length may still have an impact on recurrent restenosis. Recently, sirolimus-eluting stents have been consistently shown to reduce neointimal proliferation in in-stent restenosis as effectively as in *de novo* lesions for non-complex cases.[177] Instead of reflecting an intrinsic drug resistance, repeat restenosis in complex lesions may actually be more closely related to local mechanical conditions that impair the therapeutic effect of the device (e.g. incomplete coverage of balloon-injured areas of neointimal hyperplasia, under-expanded stents). In fact, a possible technical reason for failure was documented in 3 of 6 cases (50%) of recurrent restenosis in our series, although the significance of these findings remains elusive.

The findings from the present chapter reveal that SES for patients with failed brachytherapy is safe and is believed to be clinically effective, considering the complex population under investigation. The 0% incidence of in-hospital events as well as the absence of subacute stent thrombosis is noteworthy because the average stent length was remarkably high, and these patients are likely to have endothelial dysfunction. Nevertheless, our series indicates that the antiproliferative effect of sirolimus after brachytherapy seems to be strongly reduced compared with other situations.

In conclusion, widespread utilization of drug-eluting stents is expected to change the current scenario by reducing in-stent restenosis to a minority of

123

patients. Nevertheless, SES implantation seems to be a reasonable therapeutic option for patients with in-stent restenosis. For those with failed brachytherapy, SESs appear to be safe and are believed to be clinically effective, although our data suggest a different attenuated efficacy of sirolimus in preventing neointimal growth in this setting.

17. POST-DILATATION OF UNDERSIZED SIROLIMUS-ELUTING STENTS

Francesco Saia, Pedro A Lemos

Introduction

Several intravascular ultrasound (IVUS) studies have shown that optimal stent deployment was rarely achieved with angiographically-guided angioplasty alone.[178–180] The major effect of these studies was the introduction of routine high pressure stenting.[179–181] Moreover, stent post-dilatation with larger balloons has become common practice after the documentation of the frequent mismatch between the angiographic and the real vessel diameter,[182–184] and the very low incidence of in-stent restenosis observed in the Multicenter Ultrasound Stenting in Coronaries (MUSIC) Study with IVUS-guided stent deployment.[185] The choice to post-dilate a stent depends on many factors: operator's habit, attempt to improve suboptimal angiographic results, IVUS-guided stenting. In the Can Routine Ultrasound Influence Stent Expansion (CRUISE) study, after IVUS examination the operators decided to use oversized balloons in 34% of the patients.[186] This strategy has been proven to be safe with bare stents, and was not reported to hamper the efficacy of drug-eluting stents in the RAVEL trial,[18] where it was allowed in order to achieve a less than 20% residual diameter stenosis.

In daily practice, based on angiographic or intravascular ultrasound findings, extreme over-dilatation with balloon >1 mm larger than the stent nominal size might be required in selected cases to achieve a good procedural result. Moreover, temporary limited availability of properly sized stents could be related to local laboratory or manufacturers' problems. In sirolimus-eluting stents (SES), sirolimus is blended in a 5-μm- to 10-μm-thick layer of nonerodable polymer. Appropriate drug delivery depends on the polymer integrity and on the proper spatial distribution of the stent struts. Extreme post-dilatation of the stent could impair the effectiveness of SES in different ways: by enhancing tissue proliferation in response to greater vessel injury,[187] by altering the mechanical properties of the stent, by disrupting the polymer coating, and by increasing the distance between the stent struts, therefore reducing local drug distribution.

125

The present chapter evaluates the clinical and angiographic outcomes of patients treated with SES implantation in which a post-dilatation with largely oversized balloons was performed.

Patient population and procedural characteristics

In a four-month period of enrolment in RESEARCH, 68 consecutive patients underwent SES implantation and further post-dilatation with balloons >1 mm larger than the stent nominal size and comprise the present study population. Around 15% of the patients had diabetes mellitus, and 56% multivessel coronary disease (Table 17.1). Acute myocardial infarction was the presentation syndrome in 23.5%. Overall, 75 lesions were treated with 101 sirolimus-eluting stents, with an average stent length per lesion of 26.9±18.0 mm. Among the lesions, 7 (9.3%) were in the left main, and 9 (12%) in a saphenous vein graft. Chronic total occlusions (>3 months) accounted for 24% of the procedures. Nominal stent diameter was 3.0 mm in 98 cases, 2.75 mm in 2, and 2.5 mm in 1. Further stent post-dilatation was performed with a 4.0 mm balloon in 70 lesions, and with 4.5 mm balloon in the remaining 5. Average inflation pressure was 15.9±3.6 atm. Nominal balloon to artery ratio was 1.31±0.29. IVUS was used in 21 patients (30.8%). In 85.3% of the cases, the SES was implanted to treat a *de novo* lesion, in 9.3% to treat in-stent restenosis, and in 4% to treat a guiding catheter-induced vessel dissection

Table 17.1. Baseline patient characteristics (n=68). (Catheterization and Cardiovascular Interventions. Copyright 2004.)

Age, years	60±10
Men	45 (66.2%)
Risk Factors	
Current smoker	24 (35.3%)
Diabetes mellitus	10 (14.7%)
Family history of coronary heart disease	32 (47.1%)
Clinical Presentation	
Silent ischemia	3 (4.4%)
Stable angina pectoris	30 (44.1%)
Unstable angina pectoris	19 (27.9%)
Acute myocardial infarction	16 (23.5%)
Multivessel coronary disease	38 (55.9%)
Previous myocardial infarction	21 (30.1%)
Previous coronary bypass	9 (13.2%)
Previous percutaneous coronary intervention	17 (25%)

Table 17.2. Angiographic and procedural characteristics.
(Catheterization and Cardiovascular Interventions. Copyright 2004.)

Lesions, n	75
Target coronary artery	
Left anterior descending	21 (28.0%)
Left circumflex artery	6 (8.0%)
Right coronary artery	32 (42.7%)
Left main	7 (9.3%)
Saphenous vein graft	9 (12.0%)
Lesion type	
De novo	64 (85.3%)
In-stent restenosis	7 (9.3%)
Early re-intervention	1 (1.3%)
Guiding catheter injury/dissection	3 (4.0%)
Lesion type (AHA/ACC classification)	
Type A/B1	22 (29.3%)
Type B2/C	53 (70.7%)
Thrombus-containing lesions	16 (21.3%)
Moderate/severe calcifications	9 (12.0%)
Ostial lesions	23 (30.7%)
Bifurcation stenting	4 (5.2%)
Chronic total occlusions	18 (24%)
Glycoprotein IIb/IIIa inhibitors*	26 (38.2%)
Stent per lesion, n	1.35±0.65
Stents length per lesion, mm	26.9±18.0

*percentage relative to the number of patients (68)

(Table 17.2). Glycoprotein IIb/IIIa inhibitors were used in 38.2% of the patients. The procedure was successful in 67 patients (98.5%). One patient developed diffuse distal vessel dissection after post-dilatation of the 3×18 mm SES with a 4×15 mm balloon, inflated up to 12 atmospheres, and underwent successful emergency CABG.

Clinical outcomes

During an average follow-up of 10.1±1.7 months, 3 (4.5%) patients died, 1 (1.5%) had acute myocardial infarction, and 4 patients (6%) had a target vessel revascularization (TVR), of which 3 were TLR (4.5%). The overall rate of major adverse cardiac events was 12.0%. One patient was admitted with acute large infero-posterior myocardial infarction and cardiogenic shock, which was irreversible despite positioning of intra-aortic balloon pump. A second patient died 5 months after the procedure because of end-stage renal failure. The cause

127

of death of the third patient, who died 141 days after the revascularization procedure, is unknown: he was 75 years old, diabetic, with 3-vessel disease and moderate aortic valve stenosis, and had received a SES in the proximal right coronary artery. One patient had a small periprocedural myocardial infarction (CK max=346 UI/L, MB=73 UI/L). The angioplasty was performed in a saphenous vein graft, which was totally occluded because of in-stent restenosis. Among the 4 target vessel re-interventions, only 1 was motivated by restenosis. The remaining were 1 case of emergency bypass surgery, already described, 1 early (5 days) percutaneous re-intervention caused by incomplete ostial coverage of the right coronary artery during the index procedure, and 1 case of in-stent re-dilatation driven by IVUS diagnosis of stent undersizing despite the absence of angiographic restenosis (the patient was symptomatic and presented angiographic restenosis in another lesion located distally in the same vessel, a saphenous vein graft). There were no episodes of early or late stent thromboses.

Angiographic outcomes

Angiographic follow-up was obtained in 34 patients for 39 lesions after 210 ± 29 days (range 156–309 days). As previously specified (see Chapter 2), the reasons for repeat catheterization were: elective follow-up because the patient was included in selected subgroups in 32 cases (72.7% of the 44 patients scheduled for 6-months angiography), and clinically-driven re-catheterization in 2 patients. At baseline, mean reference diameter was 3.21 ± 0.58 mm, MLD 0.86 ± 0.61 mm, percent diameter stenosis $72\pm21\%$,

Table 17.3. Paired quantitative angiographic analysis. (Catheterization and Cardiovascular Interventions. Copyright 2004.)

	Baseline	Post	Follow-up
RD, mm	3.18±0.63	3.36±0.40	3.43±0.46
MLD, mm	0.68±0.62	2.88±0.42	2.66±0.77
Diameter stenosis, %	77±22	14±9	20±21
Lesion length, mm	20.1±14.1	–	–
Acute gain, mm	–	2.22±0.73	-
Late loss*, mm	–	–	0.24±0.61
Loss index	–	–	0.13±0.34
Binary restenosis*, %	–	–	7.7%

MLD=minimal luminal diameter; RD=reference diameter
*including one total re-occlusion

and lesion length 17.9 ± 11.5 mm. Paired quantitative coronary analysis for patients with angiographic follow-up is shown in Table 17.3. Late loss was 0.24 ± 0.61 mm, with 76% of the cases in the range between -0.5 mm and +0.5 mm. Loss index was 0.13 ± 0.34. Overall, post-SES binary restenosis was observed in 3 lesions (7.7%): 2 were proximal edge restenosis, and in one patient the vessel was occluded approximately 30 mm proximally to the target lesion (Figure 17.1).

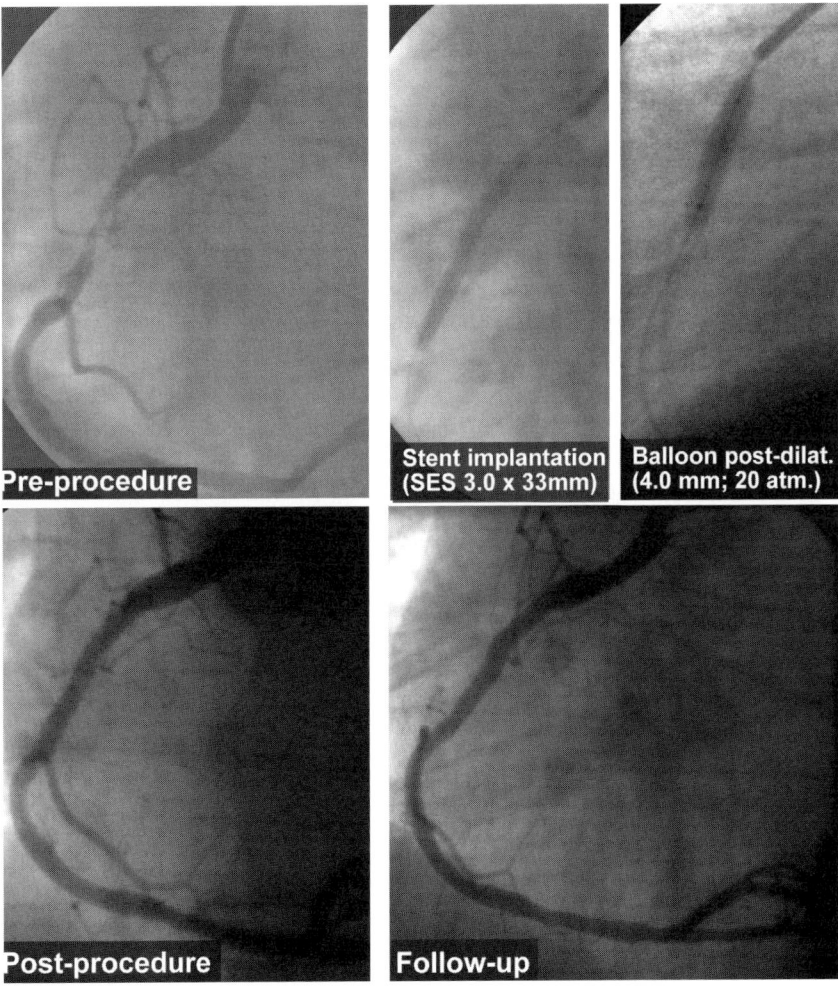

Figure 17.1 Large right coronary artery (reference diameter 4.24 mm) with a tight stenosis in its mid portion. One 3.0×33-mm sirolimus-eluting stent was implanted and post-dilated with a 4.0-mm balloon at 20 atm. The final angiographic result was maintained at 6-month follow-up.

Interpretation of the findings

The present chapter shows that post-dilatation of SES with largely oversized balloons is relatively safe and associated with good angiographic results. IVUS studies have demonstrated that incomplete stent deployment may occur in a considerable number of patients even with high-pressure techniques.[180,188] Optimal stent expansion plays a key role in the prevention of stent thrombosis.[178] Moreover, previous studies have shown that residual percent diameter stenosis after stent implantation is directly related to the development of restenosis.[3,189] Similarly, in-stent minimal lumen cross-sectional area measured by IVUS is inversely related to restenosis.[1] All together, these findings provide the rationale to pursue optimal stent expansion. This outcome is often achieved by performing stent post-dilatation with balloons oversized with respect to the nominal stent size. Over-dilatation with balloons >0.25 mm larger has been shown to improve lumen gain and possibly reduce the need for target vessel revascularization, without increasing complications.[183,184,190] However, in one study IVUS examination revealed that even with this strategy no stent reached its nominal size.[190] Thus, it is commonly believed that post-dilatation with balloons up to 0.5 mm larger than the stent nominal size can be safely accomplished in most of the cases. Conversely, dilatation with balloons >0.5 mm larger than the stent nominal size is a rare procedure. In clinical practice, this extreme post-dilatation is performed in selected patients, commonly when the operator has the perception, based on angiographic or IVUS findings, that the stent implanted is markedly undersized relatively to the vessel diameter. In other situations this choice could be driven, in a bailout procedure, by the unavailability of the proper sized stents. In both cases, this strategy should be regarded as an extreme solution, not free from potential complications.

Possible stent structure distortion and disruption must be taken into account in cases of extreme over-dilatation, as well as the chance of extensive intimal dissection and vessel wall rupture. When the same strategy is applied with drug-eluting stents, further possible shortcomings should be considered. In fact, the success of drug-eluting stents depends critically on the achievement of the appropriate local drug concentration, which warrants potent antiproliferative effects and preserved vascular healing. The elution profile/release kinetics of the drug depends on the biological properties of the drug and of the coating matrix. Apart from the potential mechanical damages to the stent, excessive SES post-dilatation could impair their antiproliferative properties by damaging the polymer coating. Moreover, by increasing the distance between the drug-carrying stent struts, over-dilatation could decrease local sirolimus concentration to a sub-optimal or ineffective level. The results

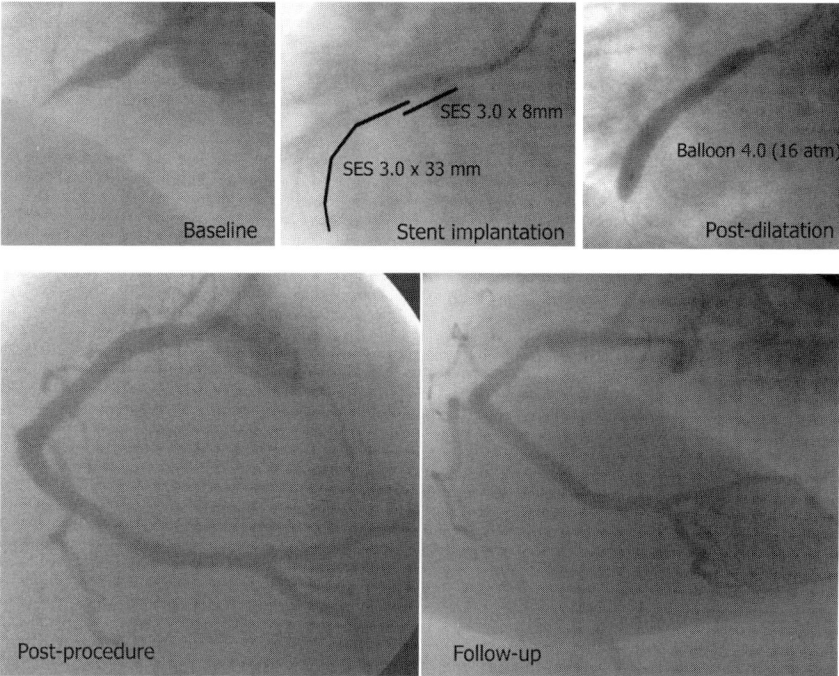

Figure 17.2 *Totally occluded right coronary artery in a patient admitted with acute myocardial infarction (upper panel, left). Two sirolimus-eluting stents were deployed (3.0 × 33 mm and 3.0 × 8 mm; upper panel mid) and post-dilated with a 4.0-mm diameter balloon at 16 atm (upper panel right). The left lower panel shows the final angiographic result (reference diameter 3.70 mm). At 6-month follow-up, there was no angiographic evidence of neointimal re-narrowing (lower panel right).*

presented in this chapter suggest that these potential risks do not have an evident impact on the favorable clinical and angiographic outcome of SES, although some negative influence cannot be ruled out in single cases. In the present series, extreme SES post-dilatation was not associated with a high rate of acute complication, although one patient had to be referred for emergency coronary surgery. The clinical outcome at mid-term follow-up was favorable, and the 12% incidence of MACE appears very satisfactory if we consider the unselected nature of the population analyzed, which included 24% of the patients with acute myocardial infarction. Notably, 9% of the lesions treated were in the left main and 12% in a saphenous vein graft. Moreover, at angiographic follow-up, restenosis was observed in a very limited number of patients. Although only 50% of the patients underwent repeat catheterization,

Table 17.4. Angiographic findings compared to the MUSIC trial (11). (Catheterization and Cardiovascular Interventions. Copyright 2004.)

	MUSIC	SES overdilatated.
Reference diameter pre, mm	3.09±0.49	3.18±0.63
Reference diameter post, mm	3.40±0.54	3.36±0.40
Reference diameter at 6 months, mm	3.04±0.51	3.43±0.46
Minimum lumen diameter pre, mm	1.13±0.34	0.68±0.62
Minimum lumen diameter post, mm	2.90±0.36	2.88±0.42
Minimum lumen diameter at 6 m, mm	2.12±0.67	2.66±0.77
Diameter stenosis pre, %	63±10	77±22
Diameter stenosis post, %	15±6	14±9
Diameter stenosis at 6 m, %	30±17	20±21
Nominal balloon/artery ratio	1.20±0.15	1.31±0.29
Maximal inflation pressure	15.8±3.33	15.9±3.6
Acute gain, mm	1.79±0.39	2.22±0.73
Late loss, mm	0.78±0.56	0.24±0.61
Loss index	0.45±0.33	0.13±0.34

the selection criteria of these patients ('complex' lesions and symptomatic patients) would have been expected to increase the chance of finding restenotic lesions, thus indirectly confirming the very positive results obtained. Remarkably, almost one fourth of the lesions were chronic total occlusions, condition traditionally associated with higher restenosis rates. Indeed, the loss index of the present series (0.13±0.34), compares favorably with the historical series of the BElgian NEtherlands Stent (BENESTENT) trial (0.46±1.39), the BENESTENT II Pilot study (0.41±1.18), and the MUSIC study (0.45±0.33) using bare stents (Table 17.4).[185]

In conclusion, angiographically or intravascular-guided post-dilatation of SES with largely oversized balloons could be considered an extreme solution for stent undersizing. Although careful case-by-case evaluation in these situations is necessary, this strategy appears relatively safe and does not seem to impair the effectiveness of sirolimus-eluting stents.

IV Complications After Sirolimus-Eluting Stents

18. THROMBOTIC STENT OCCLUSION AFTER SIROLIMUS-ELUTING STENT IMPLANTATION

Evelyn Regar, Pedro A Lemos, Patrick W Serruys

Introduction

Stent thrombosis occurs as an infrequent event after coronary stenting. However, its incidence has been largely reported to carry a high morbidity and mortality risk.[52,53,191] In the FIM study and the randomized trials reported to date,[8,12–16,18–22] stent thrombosis after sirolimus-eluting stents (SES), has occurred in only a minority of elective patients. However, after bare metal stent implantation, the incidence of sudden stent thrombosis has been previously shown to be increased in patients with acute coronary syndromes, long stents, small vessels, chronic total occlusion and multivessel intervention.[191] This chapter investigates the incidence of (sub)acute stent thrombosis (SAT) occurring in the first 12 months after the procedure in the RESEARCH population.

Study population and incidence of stent thrombosis

In the first 5 months of SES utilization during the RESEARCH, a total of 510 consecutive patients (842 lesions) were treated with 1093 SES (2.1±1.3 SES per patient) and are reported in this chapter. The baseline characteristics are shown in Table 18.1. Overall, 15.7% of patients had acute myocardial infarction and 32.4% unstable angina at admission. Multivessel stent implantation was performed in 25%, stents with small nominal diameter (2.5 or 2.25 mm) were implanted in 25.7%, and a long stented segment (> 36 mm) was recorded in 17.5%. Glycoprotein IIb/IIIa inhibitors were used in 24% of cases.

Thrombotic stent occlusion was angiographically documented as a complete occlusion (TIMI flow 0 or 1) or a flow limiting thrombus (TIMI flow 1 or 2) of a previously successfully treated artery (TIMI flow 3 immediately after stent placement and percent in-lesion diameter stenosis <30%). Acute was defined as occurring <24 hours, subacute as occurring >24 hours to <30 days following the study procedure. Late was defined as occurring >30 days after the index procedure.

Table 18.1. Baseline and Procedural Characteristics (n=510)	
Age	61.4±11.6 years
Male sex	70.2%
Diabetes	18.6%
Current smoking	32.8%
Hypertension	43.8%
Previous MI	30.3%
Previous PCI	25.5%
Previous CABG	10.0%
Previous brachytherapy	2.7%
Coronary artery disease	
Single-vessel disease	45.7%
Double-vessel disease	27.9%
Triple-vessel disease	24.6%
Stable angina	51.9%
Unstable angina	32.4%
Acute MI	15.7%
IIB/IIIA inhibitors	24.0%
Treated vessel	
LMC	3.6%
LAD	56.8%
LCx	32.1%
RCA	34.7%
Multivessel SES implantation	25.0%
Number of SES per procedure	2.1±1.3 stents
Total length of the implanted stents	38±27 mm/patient (range 8–184 mm)
Overlapping stents	52.8%
Adjacent stented length > 36 mm	17.5%
Small stent diameter (2.5 or 2.25 mm)	25.7%
Postdilatation performed	53.0%
IVUS use	20.6%
Maximum pressure	17.2±3.0 atm
Reference diameter	2.67±0.55 mm
MLD pre	0.74±0.53 mm
DS pre	70.6±19.8%
MLD post	2.28±0.54 mm
DS post	16.8±11.5%

CABG=coronary artery bypass graft; LAD=left anterior descending; LCx=left circumflex; LM=left main; MI=myocardial infarction; MLD=minimal luminal diameter; PCI=percutaneous coronary intervention; RCA=right coronary artery; SES=sirolimus-eluting stent, IVUS=intravascular ultrasound imaging

During the first 12 months after the procedure, 2 patients (0.4%) developed SAT and are detailed in Figures 18.1 and 18.2. Stent thrombosis occurred at 6 hours and 11 days after SES implantation and none of the patients died as a consequence of the thrombotic event. Both patients were diabetic females with complex coronary lesions. Moreover, they were on

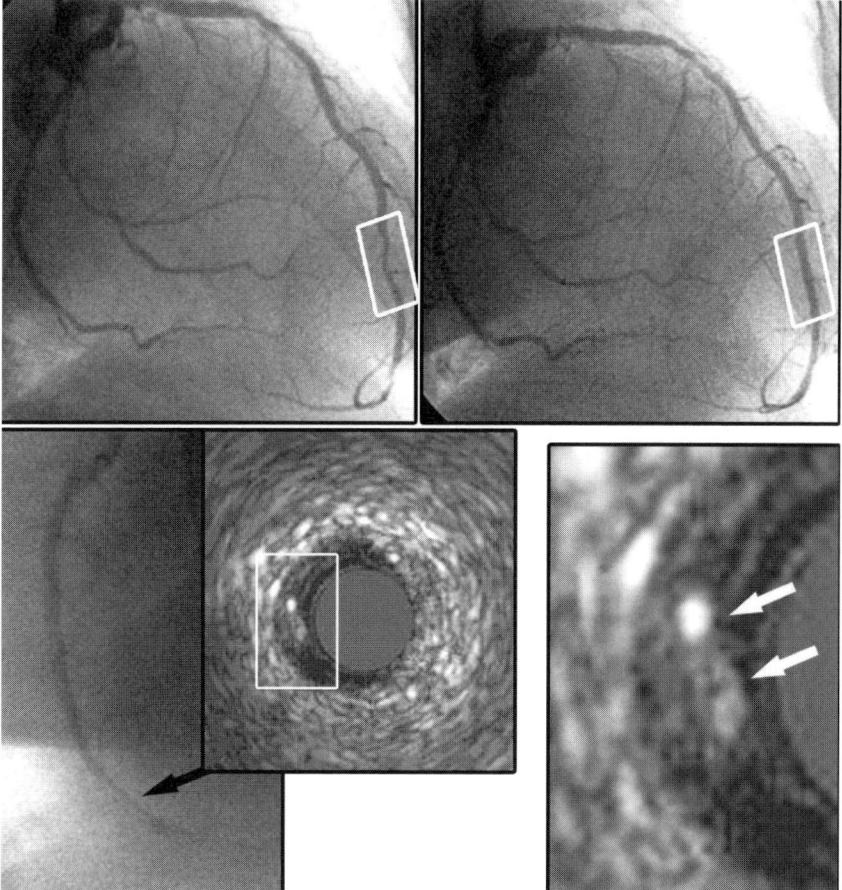

Figure 18.1 *Stent thrombosis (case 1): Pre-intervention angiogram showed a luminal narrowing located at the distal left anterior descending artery (left upper panel), which was treated with implantation of a 2.25 × 8 mm sirolimus-eluting stent (right upper panel). The left inferior panel depicts a coronary angiography obtained 6 h after the index procedure, showing total occlusion of the stent. Intravascular-ultrasound examination at the occlusion site (black arrow) showed under-expansion of the stent (minimal in-stent area 2.0 mm²; proximal reference 3.8 mm²; distal reference 3.1 mm²) (mid lower panel). Also, a distal edge dissection, which was not visible on the angiogram at the time of the index procedure, was detected (right lower panel, white arrow). (Modified from Regar et al.[191a] With permission from Excerpta Medica, Inc.)*

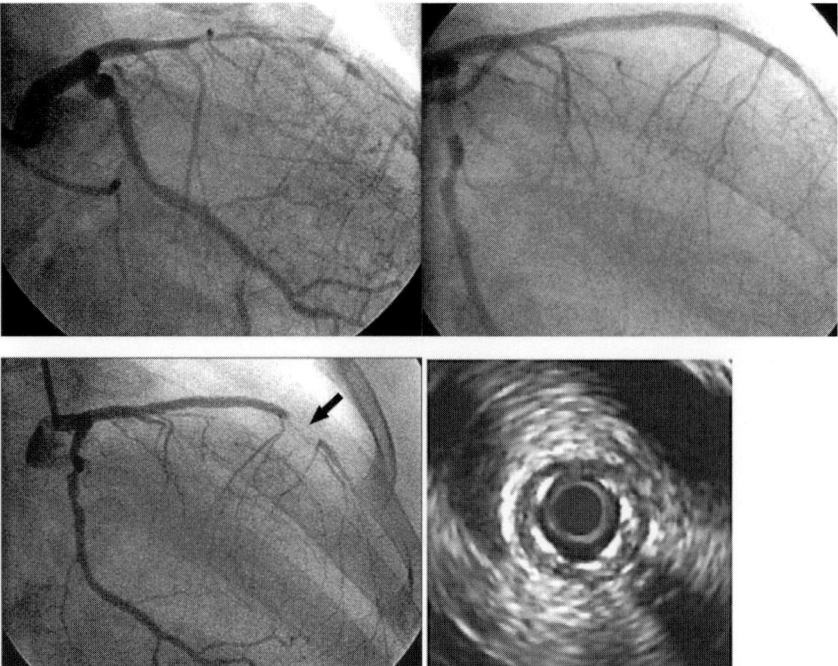

Figure 18.2 *Stent thrombosis (case 2): Pre-intervention angiogram (left upper panel) showed chronic total occlusion of the left anterior descending artery (vessel visualized by collateral filling during simultaneous contrast injection in the left and right coronary arteries). The right upper panel shows the final result after recanalization and implantation of two sirolimus-eluting stents (3.0 × 33 mm and 2.5 × 33 mm). Thrombotic stent occlusion was diagnosed at a coronary angiogram 11 days after the index procedure (left lower panel). Intravascular ultrasound examination at the site of the occlusion (black arrow) revealed an under-expansion of the stent (minimal stent area 2.27 mm^2; proximal reference 8.55 mm^2; distal reference 2.54 mm^2) (right lower panel). (Modified from Regar et al.[191a] With permission from Excerpta Medica, Inc.)*

therapy with aspirin and clopidogrel at the time of the event. In these two cases IVUS examination revealed mechanical factors that had possibly predisposed to the complication (inadequate stent expansion and uncovered distal dissection).

Interpretation of the findings

The present results revealed that SAT after SES in unselected patients occurs as a rare event, which is commonly associated with mechanical local conditions.

Moreover, no case of late stent thrombosis (>1 month) was observed. The 0.4% incidence is low and comparable to that previously reported for conventional bare metal stents. Both patients with stent thrombosis were diabetics with complex coronary lesions, which is also in line with recent findings in a large series of bare metal stents. SAT was previously found to be mainly related to inadequate post-procedure lumen dimensions or procedure-related abnormal lesion morphologies (dissection, thrombus, or tissue prolapse). Stents in the left anterior descending artery have also been reported to be more often involved in stent thrombosis than other vessels, although diameters of the left anterior descending are usually smaller than in the right coronary artery (which may per se predispose to SAT).[192]

While diabetes is a well-established predictor of adverse outcome,[8] the impact of gender is controversial. In recent studies comparing the outcome for women and men after with bare metal stent implantation, a higher event rate,[193] a lower event rate[194] or similar event rates[195] have been reported in women as compared to men.

Combined oral antiplatelet therapy[196] and systematic high-pressure stent implantation[197] have contributed to reduce the incidence of thrombotic occlusion after conventional coronary stenting. Owing to the fact that SES have virtually the same physical properties as bare metal stents, similar technical approaches were utilized in the present series to accomplish optimum SES deployment. The average implantation pressure was 17 atmospheres and balloon post-dilatation was performed in approximately half of the cases. All patients were maintained under dual antiplatelet treatment.

Previous studies suggested that sirolimus could significantly enhance agonist-induced platelet aggregation[41] and induce endothelial function impairment.[38] Animal models showed focal remnants of residual fibrin deposition adjacent to the struts that may reflect a delay in arterial repair or simply impaired fibrin degradation secondary to the local effects of the drug.[11] However, although these features could potentially increase the risk of thrombotic complications, our findings suggest a minimal risk of SAT after SES implantation, even in patients with well-known risk factors for short-term thrombotic complications.

In summary, during 12 months follow-up sirolimus-eluting stents showed a low incidence of stent thrombosis of 0.4%, which is comparable to data previously reported for bare metal stents.

19. MORPHOLOGY AND MECHANISMS OF RESTENOSIS AFTER SIROLIMUS-ELUTING STENTS

Pedro A Lemos, Francesco Saia

Introduction

Restenosis after sirolimus-eluting stent (SES) implantation occurs in a small though sizeable proportion of cases. In the RAVEL trial,[18] no cases of restenosis were seen. In the SIRIUSs trials, however, which involved lesions of higher complexity, restenosis did occur in a number of cases.[19–21] In these latter studies, post-SES restenosis has been observed to occur either at the edges of the stent or within the stent itself. In the SIRUS trial,[19] from a total post-SES restenosis rate of 8.9%, most of the restenoses occurred at the edges of the stent (5.7% at the edges and 3.2% in-stent), with the proximal border being more frequently restenotic than the distal one. Also, in the C-SIRIUS trial,[21] no cases of post-SES restenosis were observed within the stented area, whilst 2.3% of the cases had restenosis at the stent edge. Conversely, in the recent E-SIRIUS trial,[20] a predominance of edge post-SES restenosis was not observed. Instead, the total restenosis rate after SES implantation was 5.9%, of which 3.9% occurred inside the stent area. Moreover, in a preliminary report from a consecutive series of cases, Colombo et al have shown that most post-SES occurred as focal or multifocal lesions inside the stent.[198] Recently, Fujii et al observed that stent underexpansion may be a significant cause of recurrent restenosis after SES implantation treatment of in-stent restenosis.[199] Nevertheless, the morphology and possible associated mechanisms of post-SES restenosis have been poorly described.

This chapter describes in detail the main features of a consecutive series of restenosis occurring after SES implantation in RESEARCH.

Patient population and post-SES description

By February 2003 (11 months after commencing SES implantation in RESEARCH), a total of 19 patients were diagnosed with 20 post-SES restenosis lesions and are reported in this chapter (Table 19.1).

Table 19.1 Clinical, procedural, and morphological characteristics of patients with restenosis after sirolimus-eluting stent implantation

Age, years	56±11
Male	89%
Diabetes	37%
Symptoms/ischemia at follow-up	58%
Patients with other lesions treated at the index procedure that were not restenotic	68%
Vessel	
Right coronary artery	20%
Right postero-lateral branch	5%
Left anterior descending	30%
Diagonal branch	20%
Left circumflex	15%
Saphenous vein graft	10%
Treatment of previous in-stent restenosis*	25%
Moderate / severe calcification	25%
Chronic total occlusion	35%
Trauma outside the stent/residual dissection	83%†
Residual edge lesion‡	33%†
Post-dilatation with balloon ≥ 0.5 mm larger	45%
Bifurcation stenting	35%
Ostial	30%
Stented length >33 mm	40%
2.25-mm diameter SES	15%
Stent fracture or gap between stents§	50% ‖
Stent underexpansion at restenosis site§	25% ‖
Post-SES restenosis characteristics	
Location	
Total occlusion	10%
Focal lesion (length <10 mm)	86%¶

*2 of 5 of the restenotic lesions at the index procedure were failed brachytherapy lesions
†relative to proximal edge restenosis
‡angiographic diameter stenosis >30% or IVUS plaque burden >50%
§ diagnosed by IVUS
‖ relative to the number of in-stent restenosis with available IVUS
¶ relative to the number of in-stent restenosis

In total, 6 lesions (30%) were located at the proximal edge and 14 were *in-stent* (70%). Local injury outside the stent was observed in 5 edge restenosis (83%), as evidenced by the presence of angiographic or IVUS residual dissection after the procedure. Among the 14 *in-stent* lesions, 12 (86%) presented a peculiar angiographic pattern manifested by a very localized lesion bordered by segments without evidence of lumen compromise ('spot restenosis') (Figure 19.1). Lesion length decreased from 19.1±19.1 mm at

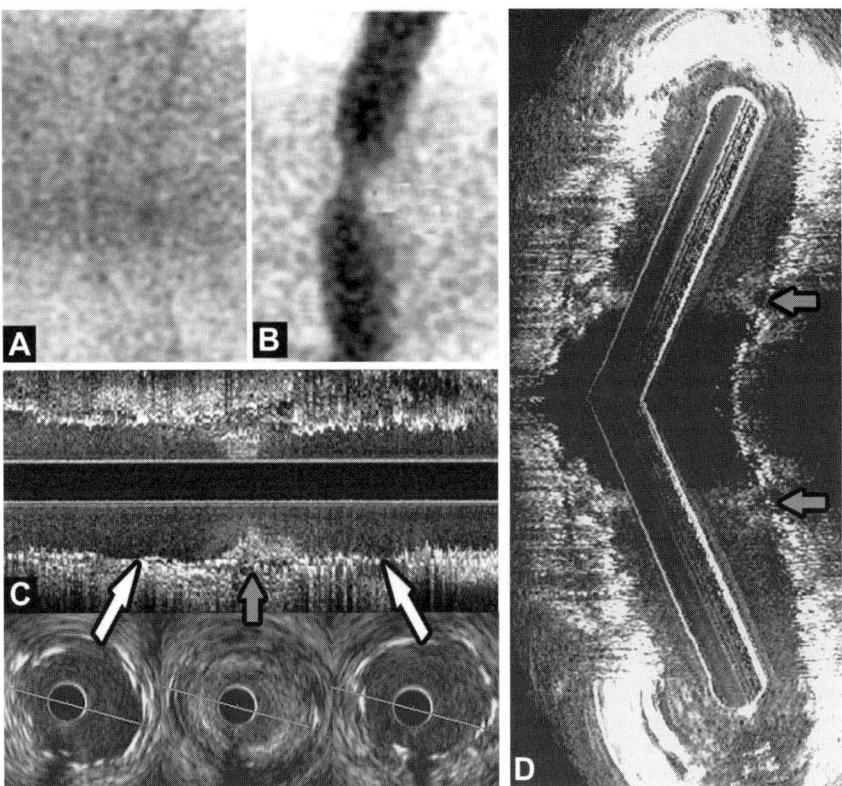

Figure 19.1 Short restenosis at the site of a small gap between stents that was not perceptible at angiography. No stent discontinuity was noted (A) at the site of luminal renarrowing (B). At intravascular ultrasound (IVUS) examination, the longitudinal and 3-dimension reconstructions showed the localized pattern of the restenosis (C and D respectively, gray arrow). The vessel circumference was covered by stent struts at the proximal and distal segments, with no evidence of neointimal tissue (lower panel, white arrows). In the IVUS cross section at stenotic site, however, the stent struts were not visualized (gap between stents) and there was excessive neointimal proliferation (lower panel, gray arrow). (Modified from Lemos et al.[199a])

baseline to 7.6±5.6 mm at follow-up (p=0.046), and the ratio lesion length/stent length was 0.3±0.2. A gap between stents or stent fracture at the site of the restenosis could be identified in 50% with IVUS at follow-up (n=8). In all such cases, the stent discontinuity could not be diagnosed angiographically and measured less than 1 mm in length by IVUS (Figure 19.1).

143

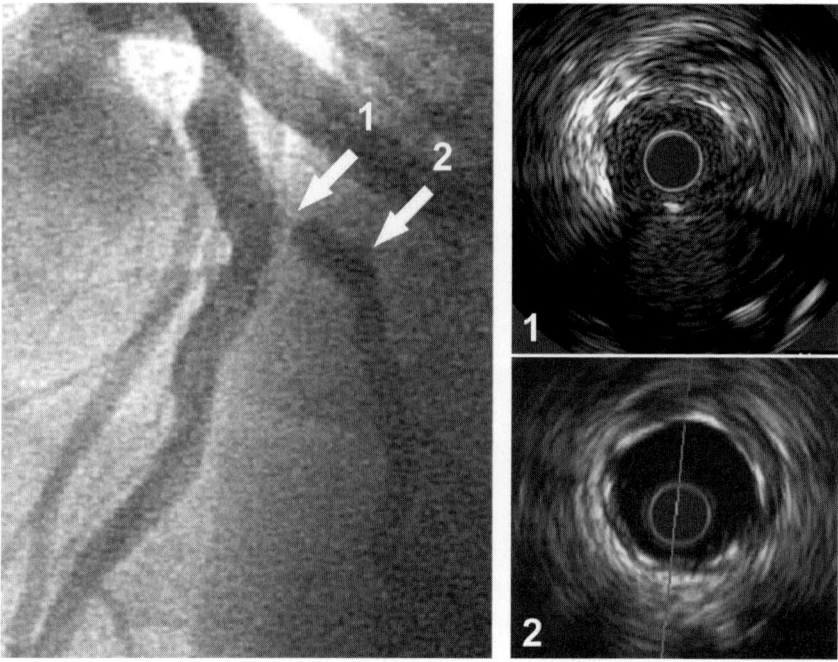

Figure 19.2 *Ostial restenosis at a site of incomplete sirolimus-eluting stent coverage. The intravascular ultrasound cross-section at the ostium (number 1) showed neointimal proliferation and paucity of stent struts, while the distal segment (number 2) showed complete stent scaffolding and absence of neointima. (Modified from Lemos et al.[199a])*

Six post-SES restenoses were located at coronary ostia (30%). At angiography, the ostium did not seem to be covered by the stent in 1 case, which was classified as proximal edge restenosis. The remaining 5 lesions appeared to be covered by stents at angiographic inspection. Unfortunately, IVUS was available for only one of these cases. However, interestingly in this case, although angiographically unnoticed, a short area at the ostium was observed to be uncovered by SES (Figure 19.2). Moreover, among the 6 ostial lesions, 4 were located in the side branch of bifurcation stenting treatment, which were all treated with 'T' stent technique (stent in the side branch implanted with its proximal border located at the ostium of the branch; stent in the main vessel implanted encompassing the side branch ostium, thereby creating a 'T' configuration).[200]

Interpretation of the findings

In approximately 90% of patients with *in-stent* restenosis post-SES, the lesion was very localized and bordered by segments with no evidence of neointima. The effect of the drug in the non-restenotic portions indicates that an intrinsic resistance to sirolimus was unlikely in most patients. Restenosis was noticed to occur frequently at the site of stent discontinuity, suggesting that a decrease in local drug availability may have contributed to the development of restenosis in these cases. Accordingly, the present findings suggest that incomplete stent coverage may also influence the occurrence of restenosis at the stent borders and at ostial sites. Although associated with high restenosis rates with bare stents, techniques that ensure complete vessel scaffold may constitute an alternative for SES implantation at bifurcations.

In conclusion, restenosis after sirolimus-eluting stent implantation may occur within or adjacent to the stent. *Edge restenosis* is frequently associated with local trauma outside the stented segment. *In-stent restenosis* occurs as a very localized lesion, associated with complex anatomy (especially ostial lesions), stent discontinuity, or diabetes. A systemic drug-resistance to sirolimus seemed to be unlikely in most patients.

145

20. PREDICTORS OF RESTENOSIS AFTER SIROLIMUS-ELUTING STENT IMPLANTATION IN COMPLEX PATIENTS

Pedro A Lemos, Dick Goedhart, Patrick W Serruys

Introduction

Several reports have previously evaluated the impact of baseline and procedural characteristics on the risk of subsequent restenosis after bare metal stent implantation, with a number of high-risk parameters, such as diabetes, lesion length, and vessel size, being consistently identified in most studies.[1–3,35,128,201,202] Unfortunately, these characteristics are commonly found in daily practice, where treatment of patients with complex lesions frequently appears as a challenging therapeutic dilemma. In the present chapter, highly complex patients treated with sirolimus-eluting stent (SES) in the RESEARCH were evaluated for the presence of post-SES restenosis. The value of clinical, angiographic, and procedural factors in predicting the risk of restenosis in this population is evaluated.

Patient population

The patient selection for protocol-mandated angiographic follow-up in RESEARCH is detailed in Chapter 3. Briefly, angiographic re-evaluation was obtained for patients with

(1) Treatment of acute myocardial infarction
(2) Treatment of in-stent restenosis,
(3) Utilization of very small sirolimus-eluting stent (2.25-mm nominal diameter),
(4) Treatment of left main coronary,
(5) Treatment of chronic total occlusion (more than 3 months in duration),

Table 20.1. Clinical characteristics of 238 patients and 441 lesions treated with SES implantation. (From Lemos et al.[202a])

Male sex, %	73
Age, years±SD	60±12
Hypertension, %	56
Diabetes mellitus, %	22
Insulin-dependent diabetes	6
Non insulin-dependent diabetes	16
Previous myocardial infarction, %	32
Previous bypass surgery, %	11
Previous percutaneous intervention, %	28
Multivessel disease, %	60
Clinical presentation	
Stable angina, %	54
Unstable angina, %	21
Acute myocardial infarction, %	26
Periprocedural IIbIIIa inhibitor, %	27
Treated Vessel	
Left main coronary, %	3
Left anterior descending, %	43
Left circumflex artery, %	22
Right coronary artery, %	30
Bypass graft, %	3
Chronic total occlusion > 3 months, %	8
Ostial location, %	22
Bifurcation treatment*	22
Treatment of in-stent restenosis, %	13
Number of stents implanted±SD	1.41±0.81
Overlapping, %	39
Total stented length, mm±SD	26.0±20.3
Stented length > 36 mm, %	17
Utilization of 2.25-mm SES, %	18
Reference diameter, mm±SD	2.50±0.61
Pre-procedure minimal luminal diameter, mm±SD	0.69±0.54
Pre-procedure diameter stenosis, %±SD	72.2±20.0
Lesion length, mm±SD	16.1±11.8
Post-procedure minimal luminal diameter, mm±SD	2.13±0.58
Post-procedure diameter stenosis, %±SD	17.2±11.1
Follow-up minimal luminal diameter, mm±SD	2.10±0.69
Follow-up diameter stenosis, %±SD	22.8±19.9
Late loss, mm±SD	0.04±0.49
Binary restenosis, %	7.9
In-stent, %	6.3
Proximal edge, %	0.9
Distal edge, %	0.7

SD=standard deviation; SES=sirolimus-eluting stent
*SES implantation in both the main vessel and the side branch

(6) Total adjacent stented segment longer than 36 mm, and
(7) Bifurcation stenting (sirolimus-eluting stent implanted in both the main vessel and the side branch).

In total, 238 patients (441 lesions) are reported in this chapter.

Clinical and angiographic findings

The main clinical and angiographic features of the present study group are shown in Table 20.1. Left main coronary stenting was present in 6% of patients, chronic total occlusion in 15%, initially in-stent restenosis lesion in 19%, bifurcation stenting in 21%, acute myocardial infarction at admission in 26%, very small (2.25-mm) SES implantation in 28%, and very long stenting (>36 mm) in 35%. A mean of 1.41 ± 0.81 stents were implanted per lesion;

Table 20.2. Univariate and multivariate predictors of *in-segment* restenosis after SES restenosis. (From Lemos et al.[202a])

	OR	95% CI	p-value
Univariate predictors			
Bypass graft	4.61	1.39–15.33	0.01
Treatment of in-stent restenosis	3.66	1.68–7.96	<0.01
Previous bypass surgery	3.24	1.42–7.41	<0.01
Bifurcation stenting (side branch position)	2.77	1.15–6.33	0.02
Ostial location	2.66	1.30–5.46	<0.01
Diabetes mellitus	2.54	1.24–5.21	0.01
Number of stents implanted	1.62	1.19–2.22	<0.01
Post-procedure diameter stenosis (per 10% increase)	1.55	1.14–2.10	<0.01
Total stented length (per 10 mm increase)	1.30	1.14–1.48	<0.01
Pre-procedure minimal luminal diameter	0.46	0.22–0.95	0.04
Post-procedure minimal luminal diameter	0.39	0.20–0.76	<0.01
Left anterior descending artery	0.37	0.16–0.82	0.02
Acute myocardial infarction	0	–	<0.01
Multivariate predictors			
Treatment of in-stent restenosis	4.16	1.63–11.01	<0.01
Ostial location	4.84	1.81–12.07	<0.01
Diabetes mellitus	2.63	1.14–6.31	0.02
Total stented length (per 10 mm increase)	1.42	1.21–1.68	<0.01
Reference diameter (per 1.0 mm increase)	0.46	0.24–0.87	0.03
Left anterior descending artery	0.30	0.10–0.69	<0.01

CI-confidence interval; OR=odds ratio; SES=sirolimus-eluting stent

149

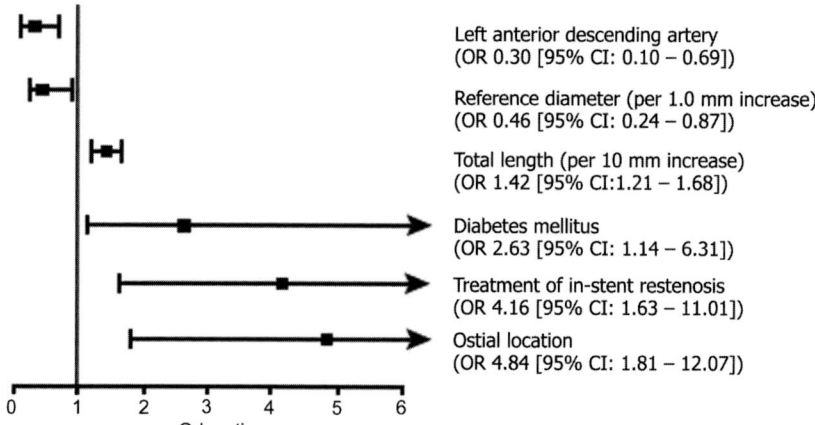

Left anterior descending artery
(OR 0.30 [95% CI: 0.10 – 0.69])

Reference diameter (per 1.0 mm increase)
(OR 0.46 [95% CI: 0.24 – 0.87])

Total length (per 10 mm increase)
(OR 1.42 [95% CI:1.21 – 1.68])

Diabetes mellitus
(OR 2.63 [95% CI: 1.14 – 6.31])

Treatment of in-stent restenosis
(OR 4.16 [95% CI: 1.63 – 11.01])

Ostial location
(OR 4.84 [95% CI: 1.81 – 12.07])

Ods ratio

Figure 20.1 *Multivariate predictors of restenosis after sirolimus-eluting stent implantation in complex patients.*

39% of lesions had at least overlapped stents. The mean vessel size was 2.50±0.61 mm (range 1.00–4.59 mm), and the average stented length was 26.0±20.3 mm (range 8–117 mm)

At follow-up, 7.9% of lesions had binary *in-segment* restenosis: 6.3% were located inside the stent (*in-stent*), 0.9% were located in the proximal edge, and the remaining 0.7% occurred at the distal edge. Significant univariate and multivariate predictors are shown in Table 20.2. In the multivariate analysis, the following variables were identified as independent predictors: treatment of in-stent restenosis, ostial location, diabetes mellitus, total stented length, reference diameter, and left anterior descending artery (Figure 20.1).

Interpretation of the findings

Binary restenosis after sirolimus-eluting stents in highly complex patient population was detected in only a minority of cases (7.9% of lesions). For comparison, based on previous prediction equations derived from studies with conventional stents, the calculated expected restenosis rate for *de novo* lesions included the present report would range from 40.1% to 43.0%, if treated with bare metal stents (Figure 20.2).[2,202]

In the SIRIUS trial, small vessel size, long lesion length, and diabetes have been shown to significantly increase the incidence of restenosis after sirolimus-

150

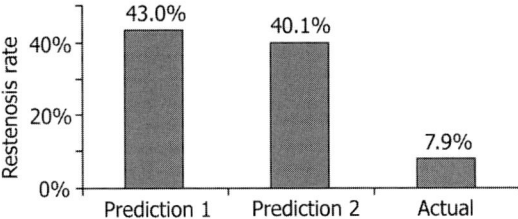

Figure 20.2 *Theoretical restenosis rates for patients included in the RESEARCH in case of treatment with bare metal stents, as calculated from predictive formulas previously reported.[2,202] The predicted incidence of restenosis with bare stents (43.0% and 40.1%) are compared with the actual data with sirolimus-eluting stents from the RESEARCH (7.9%).*

eluting stent.[19] These characteristics were confirmed as predictors of post-SES restenosis in RESEARCH, which additionally extended the list of independent parameters to also include ostial location and treatment of in-stent restenosis (as negative factors) and left anterior descending artery location (as a protective factor). Interestingly, most characteristics identified as predictors of post-sirolimus-eluting stent restenosis have long been recognized as major predictors of restenosis following balloon angioplasty or conventional bare stent implantation.[1–3,35,128,201–205] It seems intuitive to assume that the increased incidence of restenosis after SES in patients with these risk factors may reflect an extreme background tendency to tissue reaction and neointimal growth, which was not sufficiently inhibited by the antiproliferative action of the drug.

In the present chapter, it is shown that lesions involving ostial sites had a higher risk of restenosis. This may be, at least partially, related to technical difficulties in positioning the stent to ensure complete vessel scaffolding at the ostium. Similar findings were also observed in a recent study evaluating SES for bifurcation lesions, where in most cases the restenosis occurred at the side branch ostium and were focal.[151] One may speculate that the presence of 'traditional' risk factors for restenosis may potentially act as a predisposing factor, which will lead to restenosis in case a subtle device-related or procedure-related local failure is eventually superimposed. Unfortunately, small gaps between stents and minor ruptures in the metallic stent mesh or in the polymer integrity are not detectable by conventional coronary angiography and could not be evaluated.

The treatment of in-stent restenosis with SES was associated with a greater than 4-fold increase in the risk of restenosis after adjustment for other independent variables. Although SES implantation has been associated with low

151

rates of repeat restenosis after treatment of non-complex in-stent restenosis,[31,32] the efficacy of this device for more complicated cases remains to be established.[31] Re-dilatation of restenotic lesions (i.e. exposure to 'double injury') has been previously shown to trigger a peculiar local vascular response, distinct from that observed after the first dilatation.[206] Modifications in the reparative mechanisms, especially after endovascular brachytherapy, may decrease the responsiveness of restenotic lesions to the antiproliferative drug (see Chapter 16).

Importantly, post-SES restenosis was not detected in any patient admitted with acute myocardial infarction. Also, it was almost entirely restricted to the segment inside the stent (approximately 80% of the restenoses). In RESEARCH, all operators were strongly advised to actively cover the entire injured vessel area and to avoid residual dissection at the stent borders and gaps between stents. In addition, the stent placement strategy aimed to cover the treated segment 'from healthy tissue to healthy tissue', in order to avoid the free borders of the stents to terminate in grossly diseased segments. However, it remains speculative whether these procedural strategies might have had any impact in reducing the incidence of restenosis at the stent edges.

In conclusion, angiographic restenosis after sirolimus-eluting stent implantation in complex patients is an infrequent event (7.9% of lesions), occurring mainly in association with local, lesion-based characteristics and diabetes mellitus.

21. LATE LUMINAL LOSS RESPONSE PATTERN AFTER SIROLIMUS-ELUTING STENT IMPLANTATION OR CONVENTIONAL STENTING

Pedro A Lemos, Ron T Van Domburg,
Patrick W Serruys

Introduction

Several cutoff criteria have been proposed over the last decades to dichotomize patients with and without restenosis. However, it has been widely recognized that, to some extent, late luminal reduction is an ubiquitous phenomenon that occurs even for lesions classified as not restenotic according to binary definitions.[207,208] In the present study, the pattern of late luminal loss following sirolimus-eluting stents is analyzed in comparison with conventional bare metal stent implantation.

Patient population

A total of 238 patients (441 lesions) had late angiographic follow-up in RESEARCH, as detailed in Chapters 3 and 20. In the present chapter, patients treated with SES from the RESEARCH are compared with 526 patients (734 lesions) treated with conventional stents in the Evaluation of Oral Xemilofiban in Controlling Thrombotic Events (EXCITE) trial.[209]

Patients treated with SES had a higher risk profile for restenosis than the control group with bare stents, according to previously proposed risk factors. In the sirolimus group lesion length was longer (16.1±11.8 mm vs. 10.0±7.5 mm; p<0.01), the reference vessel diameter was smaller (2.50±0.61 mm vs. 2.80±0.59 mm; p<0.01), and post-procedural minimal luminal diameter were smaller (2.13±0.58 mm vs. 2.43±0.54 mm; p<0.01). Also, diabetes tended to be more prevalent among patients treated with sirolimus stents (22% vs. 17%; p=0.1).

Angiographic findings

Even though SES-treated patients were at higher risk of restenosis, the total binary restenosis rate was significantly lower (7.9% vs. 26.0%; p<0.01) and the overall late lumen loss significantly smaller (0.04±0.49 mm vs. 0.80±0.61 mm; p<0.01) in the sirolimus group than in the bare group.

Overall, patients treated with bare stents or SES had an average late loss of 0.80 mm vs. 0.04 mm (p<0.01). Lesions were then grouped as restenotic or non-restenotic according to binary definitions (DS>50%; analyses for other previously described definitions[210–212] yielded similar results). The mean late loss of restenotic lesions among controls (26.0% of lesions) was 1.40±0.64 mm and the mean late loss for SES restenotic lesions (7.9%) was 1.16±0.76 mm (p=0.02).

Non-restenotic lesions in the bare stent group presented a frequency distribution of late loss close to normality (p=0.3 by Kolmogorov–Smirnov test for normality), with an average late loss of 0.58±0.44 mm. However, non-restenotic lesions in SES presented a mean late loss close to zero (–0.05 mm with a standard deviation of 0.33 mm) and a frequency distribution also close to normality (p=0.5 by Kolmogorov–Smirnov test for normality).

Previous studies from our institution have evaluated the repeatability of quantitative angiographic measurements from acquisitions performed at the beginning and at the end of the catheterization (i.e. images were acquired within an interval of some minutes, but the X-ray system had to be repositioned to the same projection after being moved to acquire other views).[29,213] The average difference between both measurements was reported to be 0.03 mm (medium-term repeatability accuracy) with a standard deviation of 0.18 mm (medium-term repeatability precision).[29,213] The calculations performed to assess accuracy and precision in this context are the same as those used for late loss and its standard deviation respectively. Of note, the late loss and standard deviation of lesions without binary restenosis in the sirolimus group (and not in the bare stent group) were similar to the accuracy and precision of repeated measurements of the same vessel segment. These findings suggest that the values of late loss for lesions with no restenosis after SES implantation may potentially reflect solely the variability of repeated measurements, with a minimal (or absent) component due to actual neointimal accumulation (or vessel enlargement). Conversely, even when not classified as restenotic according to binary criteria, lesions treated with bare stents did present some extent of luminal loss, implying that mild neointimal proliferation may be present also in non-restenotic lesions after conventional stenting.

To evaluate this hypothesis further, repeated measurements were performed in a random sample of 30 vessel segments from our series. The repeated measurements for vessel diameters differed by –0.02 mm (repeatability accuracy) with a standard deviation of 0.29 mm (repeatability precision). The resemblance between the analyses for repeated measurements and late loss in the sirolimus stents (mean –0.05 mm with a standard deviation of 0.33 mm) was evident and clearly differed from the bare stents (mean 0.58 mm with a standard deviation of 0.44 mm).

Interpretation of the findings

The possibility of a biological all-or-none response of restenosis following sirolimus-eluting stent implantation is raised by the present findings: substantial luminal renarrowing occurred in a minority of lesions diagnosed as restenotic, according to binary definitions. In most patients, however, luminal dimensions were maintained, with zero late loss at follow-up. Moreover, in the latter group, eventual differences in luminal measurements between post-stenting and follow-up resembled variations that were expected to occur in repeated angiographic measurements. Altogether, this pattern of late angiographic outcome differed from that observed after bare stent implantation. After conventional stenting, the late loss of non-restenotic lesions in bare stents (adjusted estimate 0.58 mm) was significantly higher than in non-restenotic sirolimus stents, for which late loss was maintained close to zero.

It has been reported that some degree of late loss occurs even for non-restenotic lesions after percutaneous interventions with bare stents.[207,208] Sirolimus-eluting stent implantation, however, has been shown in the present chapter to virtually abolish neointimal formation in non-restenotic lesions. The elimination of neointima creates a peculiar scenario, in which the angiograms of non-restenotic lesions obtained immediately post-procedure and at follow-up are usually indistinguishable (Figures 21.1 and 21.2). In this context, the measurements performed to calculate the late loss (i.e. the difference in luminal diameters between both angiograms) actually mimic repeated measurements of the 'same' angiogram, a fact that is readily appreciated by the average 'late loss' of almost zero. Moreover, the standard deviation of late loss measurements (0.3 mm) represent the normal fluctuations of repeated measurements performed in the same segment. Interestingly, similar findings were observed in the FIM and RAVEL studies, where all cases were free of restenosis. In the FIM study,[13] 'late loss' was 0.16±0.3 mm (slow release formulation), while in the RAVEL trial 'late loss' was reported to be –0.01±0.33 mm.[18,136]

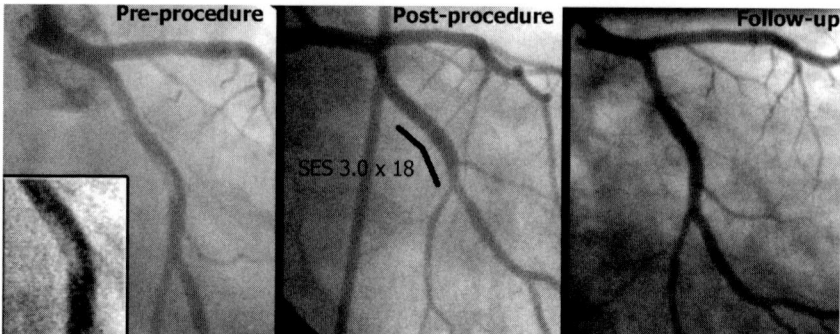

Figure 21.1 *Post-procedure and follow-up angiograms of non-restenotic sirolimus-eluting stent (SES) are almost indistinguishable. A thrombotic lesion (left panel and detail at the left inferior border) was successfully treated with implantation of a 3.0 × 18 SES. The mid and right panels show the coronary angiographies obtained at post-procedure and at 6-month angiograms respectively. The angiograms at both time points look remarkably similar.*

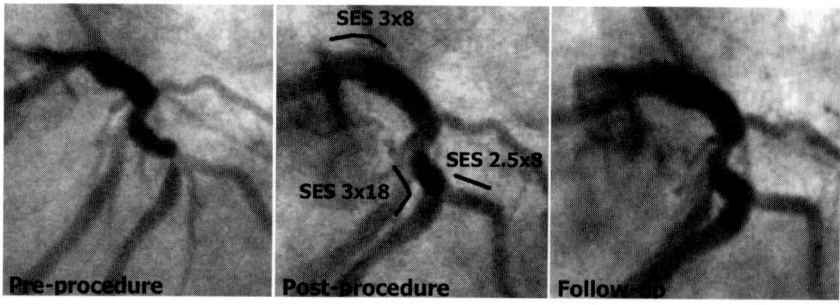

Figure 21.2 *Post-procedure and follow-up angiograms of non-restenotic sirolimus-eluting stent (SES) are almost indistinguishable. In this example, three SES were used to treat an ostial lesion at the left main coronary and at the left anterior descending/diagonal bifurcation (left panel). All stents were implanted successfully (mid panel). The right panel shows the angiogram after 7 months; all stents had a similar angiographic appearance compared to the post-procedure image, with no evidence of neointimal growth.*

In conclusion, the pattern of late loss after sirolimus-eluting stent implantation follows a peculiar behavior, which is different from lesions treated with conventional stents. The present findings raise the possibility that restenosis after sirolimus-eluting stenting may follow a biological all-or-none response.

22. TREATMENT OF POST-SIROLIMUS-ELUTING STENT RESTENOSIS

Pedro A Lemos, Carlos AG van Mieghem,
Patrick W Serruys

Introduction

Although sirolimus-eluting stents (SES) have dramatically reduced restenosis,[18–21] up to 5% of patients still need to undergo repeat revascularization. In the SIRIUS trial, it has been reported that 19 patients were re-treated with percutaneous intervention for post-SES restenosis (Dr. Jeffrey Moses, MD. Personal communication presented at the ACC meeting 2004). From these, 15 patients were re-treated with bare stent implantation, 2 with balloon dilatation, and 2 with brachytherapy (1 received an additional bare stent). The overall repeat re-intervention after treatment of SES restenosis in SIRIUS was 15.8% (3 patients).

Because post-SES restenosis is an infrequent event and the relatively recent introduction of SES in the clinical practice, little is know about the best treatment strategy for these patients. The present chapter, therefore, aims to describe the clinical and angiographic outcomes of post-SES restenosis patients re-treated with percutaneous re-dilatation.

Patient population

In the first 6 months after introduction of SES in RESEARCH, a total of 24 consecutive patients (3.8% of patients treated with at least one SES in the period) have underwent repeat percutaneous intervention for post-SES eluting stent restenosis (27 lesions) and are reported in this chapter.

Patients were treated preferably with repeat implantation of drug-eluting stents. Sirolimus-eluting stents were available up until March 2003, since then paclitaxel-eluting stents have been utilized as the default drug-eluting stent at our hospital. Nevertheless, the final interventional strategy was entirely left at the discretion of the operator. All patients receiving repeat drug-eluting stent implantation were maintained on lifelong aspirin and clopidogrel for at least 3

Table 22.1. Patient and lesion characteristics (n=24 patients, 27 lesions)

Age, years	60 (50–70)
Males, %	71
Diabetes, %	46
Multivessel disease, %	67
Treated vessel	
Right coronary artery, %	44
Left anterior descending, %	26
Left circumflex, %	15
Left main coronary, %	4
Saphenous vein graft, %	11
Ostial location, %	30
Lesion characteristics at the index procedure	
Chronic total occlusion (>1 month), %	26
Lesion type at the index procedure	
De novo lesion, %	70
Balloon restenosis, %	4
In-stent restenosis, %	15
Post-brachytherapy restenosis, %	11
Number of SES implanted at the index procedure	1 (1–3)
Total length of SES implanted at the index procedure, mm	33 (18–64)
Lesion characteristics of post-SES restenosis	
Restenosis location	
In-stent, %	93
Proximal edge, %	4
Distal edge, %	4
Lesion length of post-SES restenosis, mm	11.2 (6.6–17.1)
Treatment of the post-SES restenosis	
Balloon dilatation, %	11
Bare stent implantation, %	4
Repeat SES implantation, %	44
Paclitaxel-eluting stent implantation, %	41
Total length of repeat stent implantation, mm ‡	17 (8–30)

Numbers are medians (interquartile range) or percentages

* Related to in-stent restenosis or post-brachytherapy restenosis at the index procedure (N=7)

† Categories not mutually exclusive (intravascular ultrasound examination available for 18 lesions [67%])

‡ Related only to lesions treated with repeat stent implantation (n=24 lesions)

months. Angiographic follow-up was obtained between 7 and 10 months after the treatment of post-SES restenosis to evaluate the incidence of recurrent restenosis (>50% diameter stenosis).

158

Clinical and procedural findings

Sirolimus-eluting stents were implanted at the index procedure to treat a *de novo* lesion in 70%, in-stent restenosis or failed brachytherapy in 26%, and balloon restenosis in 4% (Table 22.1). The median length of SES implanted at the index procedure was 33 mm (interquartile range 18–64 mm). The median length of post-SES restenotic lesions was 11.2 mm (interquartile range 6.6–17.1 mm); 14 lesions (52%) were short (<10 mm long), 5 lesions (19%) were multi-focal, 7 lesions (26%) were >10-mm long, and 1 lesion (4%) presented as total vessel occlusion.

The treatment strategy for the 27 post-SES restenotic lesions was as follows:

(1) Balloon dilatation in 3 lesions (11%) (not suitable for repeat stenting);
(2) Bare stent in 1 lesion (4%) in a large saphenous graft;
(3) Repeat drug-eluting stenting for the remaining 23 post-SES restenoses (85%): sirolimus-eluting stents were implanted in 12 lesions (44%) and paclitaxel-eluting stents were used for 11 lesions (41%).

Clinical and angiographic follow-up

Clinical follow-up was available for a median period of 490 days from the index procedure and 279 days from the post-SES treatment. One patient died 412 days after the index procedure (209 days after post-SES restenosis treatment). One patient had an acute myocardial infarction which was due to subacute stent thrombosis 3 days after the treatment of the SES restenosis and was successfully treated with implantation of another SES. The treated segment was widely open at angiographic follow-up. There were no other myocardial infarctions during the follow-up period. Target lesion revascularization due to recurrent restenosis was required in 5 patients (20.8%). The event-free survival rate was 70.8%.

Angiographic follow-up was obtained for 18 patients and 21 lesions (75% of patients, 78% of lesions). The overall recurrent restenosis rate was 42.9% (9 lesions). In 3 of these cases (14.3%), the target vessel was totally occluded at the original lesion site (1 lesion) or in its proximal portion (2 lesions). An increased incidence of recurrent restenosis after treatment of post-SES restenosis was seen in patients with history of previous angioplasty (67% vs. 11%; p=0.02), previous brachytherapy at the treated site (100% vs. 33%; p=0.06), and post-SES restenosis needing treatment before 6 months from the index procedure (100% vs. 25%; p<0.01). No significant differences were

159

observed in the incidence of recurrent restenosis between short and long post-SES restenosis, and between diabetics and non-diabetics. The recurrent restenosis rate of 17 lesions re-treated with drug-eluting stents was 29.4%, with no major differences between sirolimus- or paclitaxel-eluting stents (33.3% vs. 25.0% respectively; p=1.0). For *de novo* lesions at the index

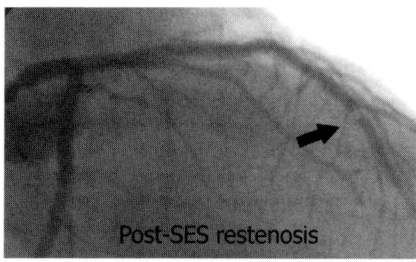
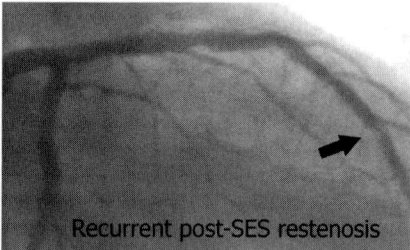

Figure 22.1 *Focal restenosis after sirolimus-eluting stent (SES) implantation (left, black arrow) in a patient with previous history of in-stent restenosis and brachytherapy at the treated site. Another SES (2.5 × 8 mm) was implanted, however the patient presented with a discrete recurrent post-SES restenosis at the same site after 10 months (right, black arrow).*

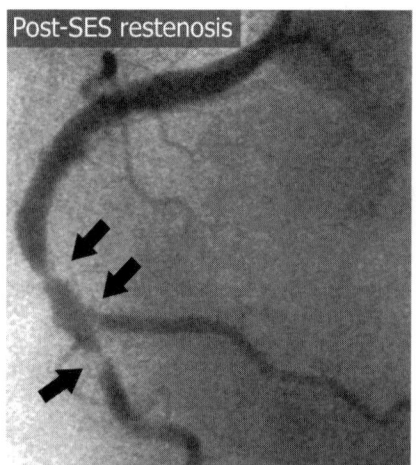
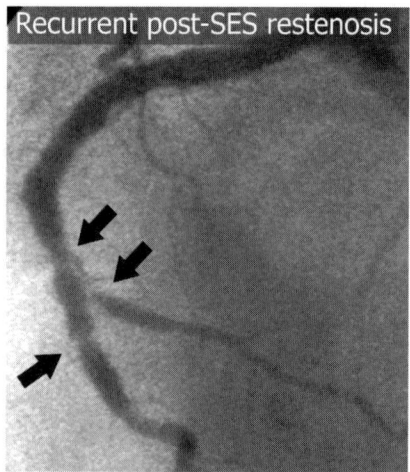

Figure 22.2 *Multifocal post-SES restenosis (Left, black arrows) in a patient who underwent bifurcation stenting using the 'crush' technique to treat a de novo lesion. The patient was re-treated with implantation of paclitaxel-eluting stents. After 6 months, the patient presented with effort angina and recurrent restenosis. Note that the pattern of the latter restenosis is similar to the former, with multifocal stenoses at the same sites seen in the first restenosis (right, black arrows).*

procedure that were re-treated with drug-eluting stents (n=11), the incidence of recurrent restenosis was 18.2% (recurrent restenosis for the remaining lesions: 70.0%; p=0.03). Two cases are illustrated in Figures 22.1 and 22.2.

Interpretation of the findings

The present results underscore the complex nature of lesions presenting with restenosis after initial SES implantation. Previous observations have shown that local features and diabetes may play an important role for a first episode of post-SES restenosis (see Chapters 18 and 19).[198] Interestingly, the presence of diabetes and the restenotic lesion length did not influence the outcomes after re-treatment in the present series. It remains speculative whether cellular mechanisms leading to drug resistance may influence the recurrence of post-SES restenosis.[214] It is worth noting that the recurrence rates were significantly increased for patients with failed brachytherapy and for those who needed early re-treatment (the latter may be related by a more aggressive restenotic process).

The main finding of the present study was that repeat percutaneous intervention for post-sirolimus-eluting stent restenosis was associated with relatively high rates of recurrent restenosis (overall 42.9%). Nonetheless, repeat drug- (sirolimus or paclitaxel) eluting stent implantation appeared to be safe, with no documented complications related to re-exposure to local antiproliferative agents. Of note, *de novo* lesions at baseline that were re-treated with drug-eluting stents had reasonably better outcomes (recurrent restenosis 18.2%), when compared to the remaining lesions.

V Costs of Sirolimus-Eluting Stents

23. COST-EFFECTIVENESS OF SIROLIMUS-ELUTING STENTS

Patrick W Serruys, Ben van Hout, Pedro A Lemos

Introduction

Sirolimus stents are sold at a high price compared to conventional bare stents, which has been perceived as an important limitation for the utilization of these devices in clinical practice. However, the reduction of repeat intervention procedures during follow-up may be cost saving, and this may eventually lower total costs. The question, therefore, arises as to how the additional effects compare to the additional costs.

The costs and effects of sirolimus-eluting stents

In the RAVEL trial, 238 patients with stable or unstable angina and a single *de novo* lesion were randomized to treatment with bare stents or sirolimus-eluting stents.[18] The effectiveness of the treatment was assessed by the incidence of major adverse cardiac events (MACE), which included all-cause death, non-fatal myocardial infarction, and target lesion revascularization (either surgical or percutaneous). With respect to costs, the analysis was limited to the direct medical costs. Sirolimus-eluting and bare stents were set with a price of €2000 and €1000 respectively. The balance between costs and effects after 12 months was assessed by computing the incremental cost-effectiveness ratio (the average 1-year costs per patient treated with drug-eluting stents minus the average 1-year costs with bare stent implantation divided by the percentage change in MACE-free survivors after 1 year).

In total, 120 patients were randomized to sirolimus-eluting-stent implantation, and 118 patients to bare metal stents. The 1-year incidence of MACE was significantly reduced in the active group compared to the controls (5.8% vs. 28.8%; p<0.01 by log-rank test), mainly due to a marked decrease in the need for repeat revascularization in the sirolimus group (0% vs. 22.9%; p<0.01). Sirolimus-eluting stent procedures were more costly at baseline (€5872 vs. €4588 respectively). However, because of the decrease in resource utilization during the first year, follow-up costs were lower for the SES group (€3473 vs. €4683). Therefore, after 1 year, the total costs for SES and bare stent patients were €9969 vs. €9915 respectively (cost difference €54). Costs per MACE-free survivor were estimated at €234 with an upper 95% limit of €5679.

It should be noted that in the RAVEL, all patients underwent protocol-mandated coronary angiography at follow-up. This may distort the incidence of events as well as the utilization of medical resources (costs) during follow-up, when compared to the usual daily practice where non-ischemia driven angiographic re-study is not commonly performed. In view of this confounding factor, an additional analysis was performed to correct the RAVEL data for the presence of follow-up angiography. Information from the BENESTENT II trial,[215] which randomly assigned patients to angiographic restudy or only clinical follow-up, was utilized for the correction in RAVEL. In this analysis, which simulated a follow-up without routine angiographic re-study, the difference in costs between the sirolimus-eluting stent and the bare metal stent at 1-year was estimated to be €166. The costs per additional MACE-free survivor are now estimated to be €1495 with an upper 95% limit of €61,243 (Figure 23.1).

In the randomized SIRIUS trial, a cost-effective analysis was performed with the stent price fixed as US$1000 and US$3000 for bare and sirolimus-eluting stents respectively (David J. Cohen, MD, MSc. Personal communication ACC meeting 2003). For this analysis, detailed medical resource utilization was collected prospectively for all patients for the initial hospitalization and for 1 year after enrolment. In addition, hospital billing data collected for index

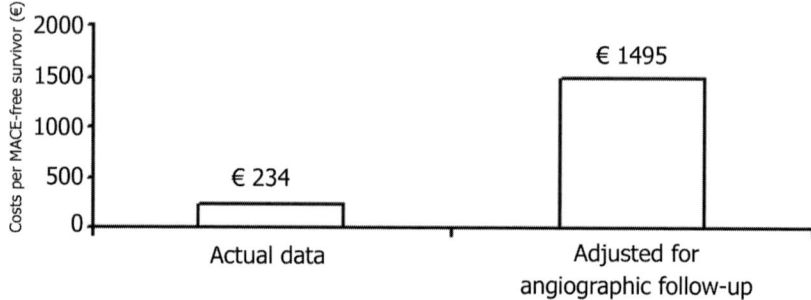

Figure 23.1 *Costs per additional survivor free of major adverse cardiac event (MACE) in the RAVEL trial. The left bar shows the costs of each additional MACE-free patient as derived from the actual data in RAVEL. The right bar shows the cost of each MACE avoided after correcting for the presence of protocol-mandated angiographic follow-up.*

admission and all subsequent admissions were obtained for 650 randomly selected patients. A regression model derived from the data of these 650 patients was used to predict the hospital and ancillary costs for the remaining hospitalizations without actual billing data collected. Costs accounted for protocol-driven angiography and non-ischemia driven TVR were excluded by the Clinical Events Committee, which was blinded to treatment assignment. The initial costs at the index hospitalization were US$11,345±3211 vs. US$8464±2497 for the SES and bare stent groups respectively (p<0.01). During follow-up, however, SES treated patients had a lower average cost (US$5468±9093) than patients receiving bare stents (US$8040±11,189; p<0.01), mainly due to a decreased incidence of repeat revascularization. After 1-year follow-up, the total medical costs for the SES and bare stent groups were US$16,813±9737 vs. US$16,504±11,511 respectively (difference +US$309; p=0.64). The estimated cost for each 'revascularization avoided' was US$1650, which compared favorably with the usually utilized 'cost-effective' threshold cost of US$10,000 per repeat intervention avoided. An additional analysis with the SIRIUS data was performed assuming availability of a more complete stent inventory (in SIRIUS, stents were available only in lengths of 8 mm and 18 mm) and equal clopidogrel use for both groups (according to the study protocol, clopidogrel should be prescribed for 3 and 1 months for SES and bare stent patients). In this analysis, SES utilization was more effective and cost-saving after 1 year (–US$96) in comparison with bare stent implantation (Figure 23.2).

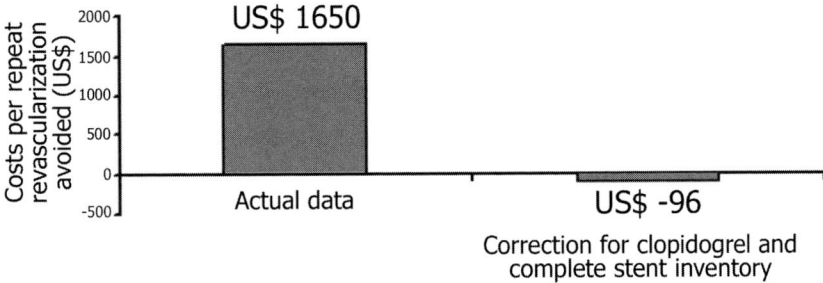

Figure 23.2 Costs per repeat revascularization avoided in the SIRIUS trial. The left bar shows the costs of each repeat revascularization avoided, as derived from the actual data in the SIRIUS trial. The right bar shows the cost of an avoided re-intervention after assuming availability of complete stent inventory (in SIRIUS, long stents were not available, which led to the use of multiple short stents in a number of patients) and equal clopidogrel usage in both groups (in SIRIUS, actual clopidogrel prescription was 1 and 3 months for bare and sirolimus stents respectively). In the latter analysis, the sirolimus-eluting stent was cost-saving; each repeat revascularization avoided 'costed' – US$96.

167

In conclusion, although drug-eluting stents constitute one of the most important advancements in interventional cardiology, costs restraints have limited their utilization in the daily practice. Nevertheless, initial analyses from randomized trials have shown a favorable cost-effectiveness profile for sirolimus-eluting stents in comparison with bare stents.

REFERENCES

1. de Feyter PJ, Kay P, Disco C, Serruys PW. Reference chart derived from post-stent-implantation intravascular ultrasound predictors of 6-month expected restenosis on quantitative coronary angiography. Circulation 1999; 100:1777–83.

2. Mercado N, Boersma E, Wijns W, et al. Clinical and quantitative coronary angiographic predictors of coronary restenosis: a comparative analysis from the balloon-to-stent era. J Am Coll Cardiol 2001; 38:645–52.

3. Serruys PW, Kay IP, Disco C, Deshpande NV, de Feyter PJ. Periprocedural quantitative coronary angiography after Palmaz-Schatz stent implantation predicts the restenosis rate at six months: results of a meta-analysis of the BElgian NEtherlands Stent study (BENESTENT) I, BENESTENT II Pilot, BENESTENT II and MUSIC trials. Multicenter Ultrasound Stent In Coronaries. J Am Coll Cardiol 1999; 34:1067–74.

4. Mehran R, Dangas G, Abizaid AS, et al. Angiographic patterns of in-stent restenosis: classification and implications for long-term outcome. Circulation 1999; 100:1872–8.

5. Braun-Dullaeus RC, Mann MJ, Dzau VJ. Cell cycle progression: new therapeutic target for vascular proliferative disease. Circulation 1998; 98:82–9.

6. Taylor AM, McNamara CA. Regulation of vascular smooth muscle cell growth: targeting the final common pathway. Arterioscler Thromb Vasc Biol 2003; 23:1717–20.

7. de Feyter PJ, Vos J, Rensing BJ. Anti-restenosis Trials. Curr Interv Cardiol Rep 2000; 2:326–331.

8. Sousa JE, Costa MA, Abizaid AC, et al. Sustained suppression of neointimal proliferation by sirolimus-eluting stents: one-year angiographic and intravascular ultrasound follow-up. Circulation 2001; 104:2007–11.

9. Sun J, Marx SO, Chen HJ, Poon M, Marks AR, Rabbani LE. Role for p27(Kip1) in Vascular Smooth Muscle Cell Migration. Circulation 2001; 103:2967–72.

10. Marx SO, Marks AR. Bench to bedside: the development of rapamycin and its application to stent restenosis. Circulation 2001; 104:852–5.

11. Suzuki T, Kopia G, Hayashi S, et al. Stent-based delivery of sirolimus reduces neointimal formation in a porcine coronary model. Circulation 2001; 104:1188–93.

12. Sousa JE, Costa MA, Sousa AG, et al. Two-year angiographic and intravascular ultrasound follow-up after implantation of sirolimus-eluting stents in human coronary arteries. Circulation 2003; 107:381–3.

13. Sousa JE, Costa MA, Abizaid A, et al. Lack of Neointimal Proliferation After Implantation of Sirolimus-Coated Stents in Human Coronary Arteries: A Quantitative Coronary Angiography and Three-Dimensional Intravascular Ultrasound Study. Circulation 2001; 103:192–195.

14. Sousa JE, Abizaid A, Abizaid A, et al. Late (Three-Year) Follow-Up from the First-in-Man (FIM) Experience after Implantation of Sirolimus-Eluting Stents. Circulation 2002; 106:II-394 [abstract].

15. Rensing BJ, Vos J, Smits PC, et al. Coronary restenosis elimination with a sirolimus eluting stent: first European human experience with 6-month angiographic and intravascular ultrasonic follow-up. Eur Heart J 2001; 22:2125–30.

16. Degertekin M, Serruys PW, Foley DP, et al. Persistent inhibition of neointimal hyperplasia after sirolimus-eluting stent implantation: long-term (up to 2 years) clinical, angiographic, and intravascular ultrasound follow-up. Circulation 2002; 106:1610–13.

17. Morice MC, Serruys PW, Costantini C, et al. Two-Year Follow-Up of the RAVEL Study: A Randomized Study With the Sirolimus-Eluting Bx VELOCITY™ Stent in the Treatment of Patients With De-Novo Native Coronary Artery Lesions. J Am Coll Cardiol 2003; 41:32A [abstract].

18. Morice MC, Serruys PW, Sousa JE, et al. A randomized comparison of a sirolimus-eluting stent with a standard stent for coronary revascularization. N Engl J Med 2002; 346:1773–80.

19. Moses JW, Leon MB, Popma JJ, et al. Sirolimus-eluting stents versus standard stents in patients with stenosis in a native coronary artery. N Engl J Med 2003; 349:1315–23.

20. Schofer J, Schluter M, Gershlick AH, et al. Sirolimus-eluting stents for treatment of patients with long atherosclerotic lesions in small coronary arteries: double-blind, randomised controlled trial (E-SIRIUS). Lancet 2003; 362:1093–9.

21. Schampaert E, Cohen EA, Schluter M, et al. The Canadian study of the sirolimus-eluting stent in the treatment of patients with long de novo lesions in small native coronary arteries (C-SIRIUS). J Am Coll Cardiol 2004; 43:1110–15.

22. Holmes DR, Jr., Leon MB, Moses JW, et al. Analysis of 1-year clinical outcomes in the SIRIUS trial: a randomized trial of a sirolimus-eluting stent versus a standard stent in patients at high risk for coronary restenosis. Circulation 2004; 109:634–40.

23. Kereiakes D, Moses JW, Leon MB, O'Shaughnessy C, Caputo RP, Kuntz RE. Durable Clinical Benefit Following CYPHER Coronary Stent Deployment: SIRIUS Study 2-Year Results. Circulation 2003; 108:IV-532 [abstract].

24. Smith SC, Jr., Dove JT, Jacobs AK, et al. ACC/AHA guidelines of percutaneous coronary interventions (revision of the 1993 PTCA guidelines. A report of the American College of Cardiology/American Heart Association Task Force on Practice Guidelines (committee to revise the 1993 guidelines for percutaneous transluminal coronary angioplasty). J Am Coll Cardiol 2001; 37:2239i–lxvi.

25. Kurlansky PA, Traad EA, Galbut DL, Singer S, Zucker M, Ebra G. Coronary bypass surgery in women: a long-term comparative study of quality of life after bilateral internal mammary artery grafting in men and women. Ann Thorac Surg 2002; 74:1517–25.

26. Herrmann C, Brand-Driehorst S, Buss U, Ruger U. Effects of anxiety and depression on 5-year mortality in 5,057 patients referred for exercise testing. J Psychosom Res 2000; 48:455–62.

27. Denollet J, Vaes J, Brutsaert DL. Inadequate response to treatment in coronary heart disease : adverse effects of type D personality and younger age on 5-year prognosis and quality of life. Circulation 2000; 102:630–5.

28. Ruygrok PN, Melkert R, Morel MA, et al. Does angiography six months after coronary intervention influence management and outcome? Benestent II Investigators. J Am Coll Cardiol 1999; 34:1507–11.

29. Reiber JH, Serruys PW, Kooijman CJ, et al. Assessment of short-, medium-, and long-term variations in arterial dimensions from computer-assisted quantitation of coronary cineangiograms. Circulation 1985; 71:280–8.

30. Moses JW, Leon MB, Popma JJ, et al. Sirolimus-eluting stents versus stsndard stents in patients with stenosis in a native coronary artery. N Engl J Med 2003; 349(14): 1315–23.

30a. Lemos PA, Serruys PW, van Domburg RT, et al. Unrestricted utilization of sirolimus-eluting stents compared with conventional bare stent implantation in the 'real world': the Rapamycin-Eluting Stent Evaluated At Rotterdam Cardiology Hospital (RESEARCH) registry. Circulation 2004; 109: 190–5.

31. Degertekin M, Regar E, Tanabe K, et al. Sirolimus-eluting stent for treatment of complex in-stent restenosis. The first clinical experience. J Am Coll Cardiol 2003; 41:184–9.

32. Sousa JE, Costa MA, Abizaid A, et al. Sirolimus-eluting stent for the treatment of in-stent restenosis: a quantitative coronary angiography and three-dimensional intravascular ultrasound study. Circulation 2003; 107:24–7.

171

33. Lagerqvist B, Husted S, Kontny F, et al. A long-term perspective on the protective effects of an early invasive strategy in unstable coronary artery disease: two-year follow-up of the FRISC-II invasive study. J Am Coll Cardiol 2002; 40:1902–14.

34. Cannon CP, Weintraub WS, Demopoulos LA, et al. Comparison of early invasive and conservative strategies in patients with unstable coronary syndromes treated with the glycoprotein IIb/IIIa inhibitor tirofiban. N Engl J Med 2001; 344:1879–87.

35. Hausleiter J, Kastrati A, Mehilli J, et al. Predictive factors for early cardiac events and angiographic restenosis after coronary stent placement in small coronary arteries. J Am Coll Cardiol 2002; 40:882–9.

36. Thel MC, Califf RM, Tardiff BE, et al. Timing of and risk factors for myocardial ischemic events after percutaneous coronary intervention (IMPACT-II). Integrilin to Minimize Platelet Aggregation and Coronary Thrombosis. Am J Cardiol 2000; 85:427–34.

37. Schuhlen H, Kastrati A, Dirschinger J, et al. Intracoronary stenting and risk for major adverse cardiac events during the first month. Circulation 1998; 98:104–11.

38. Jeanmart H, Malo O, Carrier M, Nickner C, Desjardins N, Perrault LP. Comparative study of cyclosporine and tacrolimus vs newer immunosuppressants mycophenolate mofetil and rapamycin on coronary endothelial function. J Heart Lung Transplant 2002; 21:990–8.

39. Pabla R, Weyrich AS, Dixon DA, et al. Integrin-dependent control of translation: engagement of integrin alphaIIbbeta3 regulates synthesis of proteins in activated human platelets. J Cell Biol 1999; 144:175–84.

40. Weyrich AS, Dixon DA, Pabla R, et al. Signal-dependent translation of a regulatory protein, Bcl-3, in activated human platelets. Proc Natl Acad Sci U S A 1998; 95:5556–61.

41. Babinska A, Markell MS, Salifu MO, Akoad M, Ehrlich YH, Kornecki E. Enhancement of human platelet aggregation and secretion induced by rapamycin. Nephrol Dial Transplant 1998; 13:3153–9.

42. Teirstein PS. Living the dream of no restenosis. Circulation 2001; 104:1996–8.

43. Virmani R, Farb A, Kolodgie FD. Histopathologic alterations after endovascular radiation and antiproliferative stents: similarities and differences. Herz 2002; 27:1–6.

44. Scirica BM, Cannon CP, McCabe CH, et al. Prognosis in the thrombolysis in myocardial ischemia III registry according to the Braunwald unstable angina pectoris classification. Am J Cardiol 2002; 90:821–6.

44a. Lemos PA, Lee CH, Degertekin M, et al. Early outcome after sirolimus-eluting stent implantation in patients with acute coronary syndromes: insights from the Rapamycin-Eluting Stent Evaluated At Rotterdam Cardiology Hospital (RESEARCH) registry. J Am Coll Cardiol 2003; 41(11):2093–99.

45. Wilensky RL, Selzer F, Johnston J, et al. Relation of percutaneous coronary intervention of complex lesions to clinical outcomes (from the NHLBI Dynamic Registry). Am J Cardiol 2002; 90:216–21.

46. Zaacks SM, Allen JE, Calvin JE, et al. Value of the American College of Cardiology/American Heart Association stenosis morphology classification for coronary interventions in the late 1990s. Am J Cardiol 1998; 82:43–9.

47. Cura FA, Bhatt DL, Lincoff AM, et al. Pronounced benefit of coronary stenting and adjunctive platelet glycoprotein IIb/IIIa inhibition in complex atherosclerotic lesions. Circulation 2000; 102:28–34.

48. Lindemann S, Tolley ND, Dixon DA, et al. mTOR and p38 MAP Kinase Differentially Signal the Translation of mRNAs in Activated Platelets. Circulation 2001; 104:II-223.

48a. Lemos PA, Saia F, Hofma SH, et al. Short- and long-term clinical benefit of sirolimus-eluting stents compared to conventional bare stents for patients with acute myocardial infarction. J Am Coll Cardiol 2004; 43(4):704–8.

48b. Saia F, Lemos PA, Lee CH, et al. Sirolimus-eluting stent implantation in ST-elevation acute myocardial infarction: a clinical and angiographic study. Circulation 2003; 108:1927–9.

49. Stone GW, Grines CL, Cox DA, et al. Comparison of angioplasty with stenting, with or without abciximab, in acute myocardial infarction. N Engl J Med 2002; 346:957–66.

50. Grines CL, Cox DA, Stone GW, et al. Coronary angioplasty with or without stent implantation for acute myocardial infarction. Stent Primary Angioplasty in Myocardial Infarction Study Group. N Engl J Med 1999; 341:1949–56.

51. Zahn R, Schiele R, Schneider S, et al. Decreasing hospital mortality between 1994 and 1998 in patients with acute myocardial infarction treated with primary angioplasty but not in patients treated with intravenous thrombolysis. Results from the pooled data of the Maximal Individual Therapy in Acute Myocardial Infarction (MITRA) Registry and the Myocardial Infarction Registry (MIR). J Am Coll Cardiol 2000; 36:2064–71.

52. Cutlip DE, Baim DS, Ho KK, et al. Stent thrombosis in the modern era: a pooled analysis of multicenter coronary stent clinical trials. Circulation 2001; 103:1967–71.

53. Moussa I, Oetgen M, Roubin G, et al. Effectiveness of clopidogrel and aspirin versus ticlopidine and aspirin in preventing stent thrombosis after coronary stent implantation. Circulation 1999; 99:2364–6.

54. Serruys PW, Unger F, Sousa JE, et al. Comparison of coronary-artery bypass surgery and stenting for the treatment of multivessel disease. N Engl J Med 2001; 344:1117–24.

55. Zhu MM, Feit A, Chadow H, Alam M, Kwan T, Clark LT. Primary stent implantation compared with primary balloon angioplasty for acute myocardial infarction: a meta-analysis of randomized clinical trials. Am J Cardiol 2001; 88:297–301.

56. Eisenberg MJ, Jamal S. Glycoprotein IIb/IIIa inhibition in the setting of acute ST-segment elevation myocardial infarction. J Am Coll Cardiol 2003; 42:1–6.

57. Tcheng JE, Kandzari DE, Grines CL, et al. Benefits and risks of abciximab use in primary angioplasty for acute myocardial infarction: the Controlled Abciximab and Device Investigation to Lower Late Angioplasty Complications (CADILLAC) trial. Circulation 2003; 108:1316–23.

58. Al Suwaidi J, Reddan DN, Williams K, et al. Prognostic implications of abnormalities in renal function in patients with acute coronary syndromes. Circulation 2002; 106:974–80.

59. Shlipak MG, Heidenreich PA, Noguchi H, Chertow GM, Browner WS, McClellan MB. Association of renal insufficiency with treatment and outcomes after myocardial infarction in elderly patients. Ann Intern Med 2002; 137:555–62.

60. Shlipak MG, Simon JA, Grady D, Lin F, Wenger NK, Furberg CD. Renal insufficiency and cardiovascular events in postmenopausal women with coronary heart disease. J Am Coll Cardiol 2001; 38:705–11.

61. Best PJ, Lennon R, Ting HH, et al. The impact of renal insufficiency on clinical outcomes in patients undergoing percutaneous coronary interventions. J Am Coll Cardiol 2002; 39:1113–19.

62. Rubenstein MH, Harrell LC, Sheynberg BV, Schunkert H, Bazari H, Palacios IF. Are patients with renal failure good candidates for percutaneous coronary revascularization in the new device era? Circulation 2000; 102:2966–72.

63. Szczech LA, Best PJ, Crowley E, et al. Outcomes of patients with chronic renal insufficiency in the bypass angioplasty revascularization investigation. Circulation 2002; 105:2253–8.

64. Mann JF, Gerstein HC, Pogue J, Bosch J, Yusuf S. Renal insufficiency as a predictor of cardiovascular outcomes and the impact of ramipril: the HOPE randomized trial. Ann Intern Med 2001; 134:629–36.

65. Aviles RJ, Askari AT, Lindahl B, et al. Troponin T levels in patients with acute coronary syndromes, with or without renal dysfunction. N Engl J Med 2002; 346:2047–52.

66. Gruberg L, Dangas G, Mehran R, et al. Clinical outcome following percutaneous coronary interventions in patients with chronic renal failure. Catheter Cardiovasc Interv 2002; 55:66–72.

67. Herzog CA, Ma JZ, Collins AJ. Comparative survival of dialysis patients in the United States after coronary angioplasty, coronary artery stenting, and coronary artery bypass surgery and impact of diabetes. Circulation 2002; 106:2207–11.

68. K/DOQI clinical practice guidelines for chronic kidney disease: evaluation, classification, and stratification. Kidney Disease Outcome Quality Initiative. Am J Kidney Dis 2002; 39:S1–246.

69. Dixon SR, O'Neill WW, Sadeghi HM, et al. Usefulness of creatinine clearance in predicting early and late death after primary angioplasty for acute myocardial infarction. Am J Cardiol 2003; 91:1454–7, A6.

70. Sarnak MJ, Levey AS, Schoolwerth AC, et al. Kidney disease as a risk factor for development of cardiovascular disease: a statement from the American Heart Association Councils on Kidney in Cardiovascular Disease, High Blood Pressure Research, Clinical Cardiology, and Epidemiology and Prevention. Circulation 2003; 108:2154–69.

71. Gibson CM, Pinto DS, Murphy SA, et al. Association of creatinine and creatinine clearance on presentation in acute myocardial infarction with subsequent mortality. J Am Coll Cardiol 2003; 42:1535–43.

72. Cockcroft DW, Gault MH. Prediction of creatinine clearance from serum creatinine. Nephron 1976; 16:31–41.

73. Campeau L, Enjalbert M, Lesperance J, Vaislic C, Grondin CM, Bourassa MG. Atherosclerosis and late closure of aortocoronary saphenous vein grafts: sequential angiographic studies at 2 weeks, 1 year, 5 to 7 years, and 10 to 12 years after surgery. Circulation 1983; 68:II1–7.

74. FitzGibbon GM, Leach AJ, Kafka HP, Keon WJ. Coronary bypass graft fate: long-term angiographic study. J Am Coll Cardiol 1991; 17:1075–80.

75. Kroncke GM, Kosolcharoen P, Clayman JA, Peduzzi PN, Detre K, Takaro T. Five-year changes in coronary arteries of medical and surgical patients of the Veterans Administration Randomized Study of Bypass Surgery. Circulation 1988; 78:I144–50.

76. Hwang MH, Meadows WR, Palac RT, et al. Progression of native coronary artery disease at 10 years: insights from a randomized study of medical versus surgical therapy for angina. J Am Coll Cardiol 1990; 16:1066–70.

175

77. Cameron AA, Davis KB, Rogers WJ. Recurrence of angina after coronary artery bypass surgery: predictors and prognosis (CASS Registry). Coronary Artery Surgery Study. J Am Coll Cardiol 1995; 26:895–9.

78. Foster ED. Reoperation for coronary artery disease. Circulation 1985; 72:V59–64.

79. Loop FD. A 20-year experience in coronary artery reoperation. Eur Heart J 1989; 10 Suppl H:78–84.

80. Savage MP, Douglas JS, Jr., Fischman DL, et al. Stent placement compared with balloon angioplasty for obstructed coronary bypass grafts. Saphenous Vein De Novo Trial Investigators. N Engl J Med 1997; 337:740–7.

81. de Jaegere PP, van Domburg RT, Feyter PJ, et al. Long-term clinical outcome after stent implantation in saphenous vein grafts. J Am Coll Cardiol 1996; 28:89–96.

81a. Hoye A, Lemos PA, Arampatzis CA, et al. Effectiveness of the sirolimus-eluting stent in the treatment of patients with a prior history of coronary artery bypass graft surgery. Coron Artery Dis 2004; 15(3):171–5.

82. Kleiman NS, Anderson HV, Rogers WJ, Theroux P, Thompson B, Stone PH. Comparison of outcome of patients with unstable angina and non-Q-wave acute myocardial infarction with and without prior coronary artery bypass grafting (Thrombolysis in Myocardial Ischemia III Registry). Am J Cardiol 1996; 77:227–31.

83. Stone GW, Brodie BR, Griffin JJ, et al. Clinical and angiographic outcomes in patients with previous coronary artery bypass graft surgery treated with primary balloon angioplasty for acute myocardial infarction. Second Primary Angioplasty in Myocardial Infarction Trial (PAMI-2) Investigators. J Am Coll Cardiol 2000; 35:605–11.

84. Mathew V, Berger PB, Lennon RJ, Gersh BJ, Holmes DR, Jr. Comparison of percutaneous interventions for unstable angina pectoris in patients with and without previous coronary artery bypass grafting. Am J Cardiol 2000; 86:931–7.

85. Al Suwaidi J, Velianou JL, Berger PB, et al. Primary percutaneous coronary interventions in patients with acute myocardial infarction and prior coronary artery bypass grafting. Am Heart J 2001; 142:452–9.

86. Bourassa MG, Detre KM, Johnston JM, Vlachos HA, Holubkov R. Effect of prior revascularization on outcome following percutaneous coronary intervention; NHLBI Dynamic Registry. Eur Heart J 2002; 23:1546–55.

87. Garzon P, Sheppard R, Eisenberg MJ, et al. Comparison of event and procedure rates following percutaneous transluminal coronary angioplasty in patients with and without previous coronary artery bypass graft surgery [the ROSETTA (Routine versus Selective Exercise Treadmill Testing after Angioplasty) Registry]. Am J Cardiol 2002; 89:251–6.

88. Douglas JS, Jr., Gruentzig AR, King SB, 3rd, et al. Percutaneous transluminal coronary angioplasty in patients with prior coronary bypass surgery. J Am Coll Cardiol 1983; 2:745–54.

89. Morrison DA, Sethi G, Sacks J, et al. Percutaneous coronary intervention versus repeat bypass surgery for patients with medically refractory myocardial ischemia: AWESOME randomized trial and registry experience with post-CABG patients. J Am Coll Cardiol 2002; 40:1951–4.

90. Platko WP, Hollman J, Whitlow PL, Franco I. Percutaneous transluminal angioplasty of saphenous vein graft stenosis: long-term follow-up. J Am Coll Cardiol 1989; 14:1645–50.

91. de Feyter PJ, van Suylen RJ, de Jaegere PP, Topol EJ, Serruys PW. Balloon angioplasty for the treatment of lesions in saphenous vein bypass grafts. J Am Coll Cardiol 1993; 21:1539–49.

92. Lowe HC, Oesterle SN, Khachigian LM. Coronary in-stent restenosis: current status and future strategies. J Am Coll Cardiol 2002; 39:183–93.

93. Plokker HW, Meester BH, Serruys PW. The Dutch experience in percutaneous transluminal angioplasty of narrowed saphenous veins used for aortocoronary arterial bypass. Am J Cardiol 1991; 67:361–6.

94. Bhargava B, Karthikeyan G, Abizaid AS, Mehran R. New approaches to preventing restenosis. Bmj 2003; 327:274–9.

95. Keeley EC, Aliabadi D, O'Neill WW, Safian RD. Immediate and long-term results of elective and emergent percutaneous interventions on protected and unprotected severely narrowed left main coronary arteries. Am J Cardiol 1999; 83:242–6, A5.

96. Park SJ, Hong MK, Lee CW, et al. Elective stenting of unprotected left main coronary artery stenosis: effect of debulking before stenting and intravascular ultrasound guidance. J Am Coll Cardiol 2001; 38:1054–60.

97. Park SJ, Park SW, Hong MK, et al. Long-term (three-year) outcomes after stenting of unprotected left main coronary artery stenosis in patients with normal left ventricular function. Am J Cardiol 2003; 91:12–16.

98. Tan WA, Tamai H, Park SJ, et al. Long-term clinical outcomes after unprotected left main trunk percutaneous revascularization in 279 patients. Circulation 2001; 104:1609–14.

99. Takagi T, Stankovic G, Finci L, et al. Results and long-term predictors of adverse clinical events after elective percutaneous interventions on unprotected left main coronary artery. Circulation 2002; 106:698–702.

100. Prospective randomised study of coronary artery bypass surgery in stable angina pectoris. Second interim report by the European Coronary Surgery Study Group. Lancet 1980; 2:491–5.

101. Lemos PA, Cummins P, Lee CH, et al. Usefulness of percutaneous left ventricular assistance to support high-risk percutaneous coronary interventions. Am J Cardiol 2003; 91:479–81.

102. Marso SP, Steg G, Plokker T, et al. Catheter-based reperfusion of unprotected left main stenosis during an acute myocardial infarction (the ULTIMA experience). Unprotected Left Main Trunk Intervention Multi-center Assessment. Am J Cardiol 1999; 83:1513–17.

103. Chauhan A, Zubaid M, Ricci DR, et al. Left main intervention revisited: early and late outcome of PTCA and stenting. Cathet Cardiovasc Diagn 1997; 41:21–9.

104. Pocock SJ, Henderson RA, Rickards AF, et al. Meta-analysis of randomised trials comparing coronary angioplasty with bypass surgery. Lancet 1995; 346:1184–9.

105. Rodriguez A, Bernardi V, Navia J, et al. Argentine Randomized Study: Coronary Angioplasty with Stenting versus Coronary Bypass Surgery in patients with Multiple-Vessel Disease (ERACI II): 30-day and one-year follow-up results. ERACI II Investigators. J Am Coll Cardiol 2001; 37:51–8.

106. Morrison DA, Sethi G, Sacks J, et al. Percutaneous coronary intervention versus coronary artery bypass graft surgery for patients with medically refractory myocardial ischemia and risk factors for adverse outcomes with bypass: a multicenter, randomized trial. Investigators of the Department of Veterans Affairs Cooperative Study #385, the Angina With Extremely Serious Operative Mortality Evaluation (AWESOME). J Am Coll Cardiol 2001; 38:143–9.

107. Srinivas VS, Brooks MM, Detre KM, et al. Contemporary percutaneous coronary intervention versus balloon angioplasty for multivessel coronary artery disease: a comparison of the National Heart, Lung and Blood Institute Dynamic Registry and the Bypass Angioplasty Revascularization Investigation (BARI) study. Circulation 2002; 106:1627–33.

108. The SoS Investigators. Coronary artery bypass surgery versus percutaneous coronary intervention with stent implantation in patients with multivessel coronary artery disease (the Stent or Surgery trial): a randomised controlled trial. Lancet 2002; 360:965–70.

109. Kastrati A, Schomig A, Elezi S, Schuhlen H, Wilhelm M, Dirschinger J. Interlesion dependence of the risk for restenosis in patients with coronary stent placement in multiple lesions. Circulation 1998; 97:2396–401.

110. Rodriguez A, Rodriguez Alemparte M, Baldi J, et al. Coronary stenting versus coronary bypass surgery in patients with multiple vessel disease and significant proximal LAD stenosis: results from the ERACI II study. Heart 2003; 89:184–8.

111. De Gregorio J, Kobayashi Y, Albiero R, et al. Coronary artery stenting in the elderly: short-term outcome and long-term angiographic and clinical follow-up. J Am Coll Cardiol 1998; 32:577–83.

112. Kobayashi Y, Mehran R, Mintz GS, et al. Comparison of in-hospital and one-year outcomes after multiple coronary arterial stenting in patients > or =80 years old versus those <80 years old. Am J Cardiol 2003; 92:443–6.

113. Abizaid AS, Mintz GS, Abizaid A, et al. Influence of patient age on acute and late clinical outcomes following Palmaz-Schatz coronary stent implantation. Am J Cardiol 2000; 85:338–43.

114. Pfisterer M, Buser P, Osswald S, et al. Outcome of elderly patients with chronic symptomatic coronary artery disease with an invasive vs optimized medical treatment strategy: one-year results of the randomized TIME trial. Jama 2003; 289:1117–23.

115. Kahn JK. Angiographic suitability for catheter revascularization of total coronary occlusions in patients from a community hospital setting. Am Heart J 1993; 126:561–4.

116. Ruygrok PN, De Jaegere PP, Verploegh JJ, Van Domburg RT, De Feyter PJ. Immediate outcome following coronary angioplasty. A contemporary single centre audit. Eur Heart J 1995; 16 Suppl L:24–9.

117. Stone GW, Rutherford BD, McConahay DR, et al. Procedural outcome of angioplasty for total coronary artery occlusion: an analysis of 971 lesions in 905 patients. J Am Coll Cardiol 1990; 15:849–56.

118. Ivanhoe RJ, Weintraub WS, Douglas JS, Jr., et al. Percutaneous transluminal coronary angioplasty of chronic total occlusions. Primary success, restenosis, and long-term clinical follow-up. Circulation 1992; 85:106–15.

119. Sirnes PA, Golf S, Myreng Y, et al. Stenting in Chronic Coronary Occlusion (SICCO): a randomized, controlled trial of adding stent implantation after successful angioplasty. J Am Coll Cardiol 1996; 28:1444–51.

120. Rubartelli P, Niccoli L, Verna E, et al. Stent implantation versus balloon angioplasty in chronic coronary occlusions: results from the GISSOC trial. Gruppo Italiano di Studio sullo Stent nelle Occlusioni Coronariche. J Am Coll Cardiol 1998; 32:90–6.

121. Lotan C, Rozenman Y, Hendler A, et al. Stents in total occlusion for restenosis prevention. The multicentre randomized STOP study. The Israeli Working Group for Interventional Cardiology. Eur Heart J 2000; 21:1960–6.

122. Buller CE, Dzavik V, Carere RG, et al. Primary stenting versus balloon angioplasty in occluded coronary arteries: the Total Occlusion Study of Canada (TOSCA). Circulation 1999; 100:236–42.

123. Serruys PW, Hamburger JN, Koolen JJ, et al. Total occlusion trial with angioplasty by using laser guidewire. The TOTAL trial. Eur Heart J 2000; 21:1797–805.

123a.Hoye A, Tanabe K, Lemos PA, et al. Significant reduction in restenosis after the use of sirolimus-eluting stents in the treatment of chronic total occlusions. J Am Coll Cardiol 2004; 43(11):1954–8.

124. Finci L, Meier B, Favre J, Righetti A, Rutishauser W. Long-term results of successful and failed angioplasty for chronic total coronary arterial occlusion. Am J Cardiol 1990; 66:660–2.

125. Puma JA, Sketch MH, Jr., Tcheng JE, et al. Percutaneous revascularization of chronic coronary occlusions: an overview. J Am Coll Cardiol 1995; 26:1–11.

126. Rambaldi R, Hamburger JN, Geleijnse ML, et al. Early recovery of wall motion abnormalities after recanalization of chronic totally occluded coronary arteries: a dobutamine echocardiographic, prospective, single-center experience. Am Heart J 1998; 136:831–6.

127. Suero JA, Marso SP, Jones PG, et al. Procedural outcomes and long-term survival among patients undergoing percutaneous coronary intervention of a chronic total occlusion in native coronary arteries: a 20-year experience. J Am Coll Cardiol 2001; 38:409–14.

128. Kastrati A, Schomig A, Elezi S, et al. Predictive factors of restenosis after coronary stent placement. J Am Coll Cardiol 1997; 30:1428–36.

129. Olivari Z, Rubartelli P, Piscione F, et al. Immediate results and one-year clinical outcome after percutaneous coronary interventions in chronic total occlusions: data from a multicenter, prospective, observational study (TOAST-GISE). J Am Coll Cardiol 2003; 41:1672–8.

130. Park SW, Lee CW, Hong MK, et al. Randomized comparison of coronary stenting with optimal balloon angioplasty for treatment of lesions in small coronary arteries. Eur Heart J 2000; 21:1785–9.

131. Kastrati A, Schomig A, Dirschinger J, et al. A randomized trial comparing stenting with balloon angioplasty in small vessels in patients with symptomatic coronary artery disease. ISAR-SMART Study Investigators. Intracoronary Stenting or Angioplasty for Restenosis Reduction in Small Arteries. Circulation 2000; 102:2593–8.

132. Koning R, Eltchaninoff H, Commeau P, et al. Stent placement compared with balloon angioplasty for small coronary arteries: in-hospital and 6-month clinical and angiographic results. Circulation 2001; 104:1604–8.

133. Doucet S, Schalij MJ, Vrolix MC, et al. Stent placement to prevent restenosis after angioplasty in small coronary arteries. Circulation 2001; 104:2029–33.

134. Moer R, Myreng Y, Molstad P, et al. Stenting in small coronary arteries (SISCA) trial. A randomized comparison between balloon angioplasty and the heparin-coated beStent. J Am Coll Cardiol 2001; 38:1598–603.

135. Haude M, Konorza TF, Kalnins U, et al. Heparin-coated stent placement for the treatment of stenoses in small coronary arteries of symptomatic patients. Circulation 2003; 107:1265–70.

136. Regar E, Serruys PW, Bode C, et al. Angiographic findings of the multicenter Randomized Study With the Sirolimus-Eluting Bx Velocity Balloon-Expandable Stent (RAVEL): sirolimus-eluting stents inhibit restenosis irrespective of the vessel size. Circulation 2002; 106:1949–56.

136a. Lemos PA, Arampatzis CA, Saia F, et al. Treatment of very small vessels with 2.25-mm diameter sirolimus-eluting stents (from the RESEARCH registry). Am J Cardiol 2004; 93(5):633–6.

137. Kobayashi Y, De Gregorio J, Kobayashi N, et al. Stented segment length as an independent predictor of restenosis. J Am Coll Cardiol 1999; 34:651–9.

138. Kornowski R, Mehran R, Satler LF, et al. Procedural results and late clinical outcomes following multivessel coronary stenting. J Am Coll Cardiol 1999; 33:420–6.

139. Serruys PW, Foley DP, Suttorp MJ, et al. A randomized comparison of the value of additional stenting after optimal balloon angioplasty for long coronary lesions: final results of the additional value of NIR stents for treatment of long coronary lesions (ADVANCE) study. J Am Coll Cardiol 2002; 39:393–9.

140. Hoffmann R, Herrmann G, Silber S, et al. Randomized comparison of success and adverse event rates and cost effectiveness of one long versus two short stents for treatment of long coronary narrowings. Am J Cardiol 2002; 90:460–4.

141. Oemrawsingh PV, Mintz GS, Schalij MJ, Zwinderman AH, Jukema JW, van der Wall EE. Intravascular ultrasound guidance improves angiographic and clinical outcome of stent implantation for long coronary artery stenoses: final results of a randomized comparison with angiographic guidance (TULIP Study). Circulation 2003; 107:62–7.

142. Schalij MJ, Udayachalerm W, Oemrawsingh P, Jukema JW, Reiber JH, Bruschke AV. Stenting of long coronary artery lesions: initial angiographic results and 6-month clinical outcome of the micro stent II-XL. Catheter Cardiovasc Interv 1999; 48:105–12.

143. Kornowski R, Bhargava B, Fuchs S, et al. Procedural results and late clinical outcomes after percutaneous interventions using long (> or = 25 mm) versus short (<20 mm) stents. J Am Coll Cardiol 2000; 35:612–18.

143a. Degertekin M, Arampatzis CA, Lemos PA, et al. Very long sirolimus-eluting stent implantation for de novo coronary lesions. Am J Cardiol 2004; 93(7):826–9.

144. Al Suwaidi J, Yeh W, Cohen HA, Detre KM, Williams DO, Holmes DR, Jr. Immediate and one-year outcome in patients with coronary bifurcation lesions in the modern era (NHLBI dynamic registry). Am J Cardiol 2001; 87:1139–44.

145. Lefevre T, Louvard Y, Morice MC, Loubeyre C, Piechaud JF, Dumas P. Stenting of bifurcation lesions: a rational approach. J Interv Cardiol 2001; 14:573–85.

146. Brener SJ, Leya FS, Apperson-Hansen C, Cowley MJ, Califf RM, Topol EJ. A comparison of debulking versus dilatation of bifurcation coronary arterial narrowings (from the CAVEAT I Trial). Coronary Angioplasty Versus Excisional Atherectomy Trial-I. Am J Cardiol 1996; 78:1039–41.

147. Anzuini A, Briguori C, Rosanio S, et al. Immediate and long-term clinical and angiographic results from Wiktor stent treatment for true bifurcation narrowings. Am J Cardiol 2001; 88:1246–50.

148. Pan M, Suarez de Lezo J, Medina A, et al. Simple and complex stent strategies for bifurcated coronary arterial stenosis involving the side branch origin. Am J Cardiol 1999; 83:1320–5.

149. Chevalier B, Glatt B, Royer T, Guyon P. Placement of coronary stents in bifurcation lesions by the 'culotte' technique. Am J Cardiol 1998; 82:943–9.

150. Colombo A, Stankovic G, Orlic D, et al. Modified T-stenting technique with crushing for bifurcation lesions: immediate results and 30-day outcome. Catheter Cardiovasc Interv 2003; 60:145–51.

151. Colombo A, Moses JW, Morice MC, et al. Randomized study to evaluate sirolimus-eluting stents implanted at coronary bifurcation lesions. Circulation 2004; 109:1244–9.

152. Al Suwaidi J, Berger PB, Rihal CS, et al. Immediate and long-term outcome of intracoronary stent implantation for true bifurcation lesions. J Am Coll Cardiol 2000; 35:929–36.

153. Yamashita T, Nishida T, Adamian MG, et al. Bifurcation lesions: two stents versus one stent—immediate and follow-up results. J Am Coll Cardiol 2000; 35:1145–51.

154. Fuster V, Fayad ZA, Badimon JJ. Acute coronary syndromes: biology. Lancet 1999; 353 Suppl 2:SII5–9.

155. Falk E, Shah PK, Fuster V. Coronary plaque disruption. Circulation 1995; 92:657–71.

156. Ambrose JA, Tannenbaum MA, Alexopoulos D, et al. Angiographic progression of coronary artery disease and the development of myocardial infarction. J Am Coll Cardiol 1988; 12:56–62.

157. Burke AP, Kolodgie FD, Farb A, et al. Healed plaque ruptures and sudden coronary death: evidence that subclinical rupture has a role in plaque progression. Circulation 2001; 103:934–40.

158. Virmani R, Kolodgie FD, Burke AP, Farb A, Schwartz SM. Lessons from sudden coronary death: a comprehensive morphological classification scheme for atherosclerotic lesions. Arterioscler Thromb Vasc Biol 2000; 20:1262–75.

159. Arbustini E, Dal Bello B, Morbini P, et al. Plaque erosion is a major substrate for coronary thrombosis in acute myocardial infarction. Heart 1999; 82:269–72.

160. Mercado N, Maier W, Boersma E, et al. Clinical and angiographic outcome of patients with mild coronary lesions treated with balloon angioplasty or coronary stenting. Implications for mechanical plaque sealing. Eur Heart J 2003; 24:541–51.

161. Abizaid AS, Mintz GS, Mehran R, et al. Long-term follow-up after percutaneous transluminal coronary angioplasty was not performed based on intravascular ultrasound findings: importance of lumen dimensions. Circulation 1999; 100:256–61.

162. Rieber J, Schiele TM, Koenig A, et al. Long-term safety of therapy stratification in patients with intermediate coronary lesions based on intracoronary pressure measurements. Am J Cardiol 2002; 90:1160–4.

163. Ferrari M, Schnell B, Werner GS, Figulla HR. Safety of deferring angioplasty in patients with normal coronary flow velocity reserve. J Am Coll Cardiol 1999; 33:82–7.

164. Bech GJ, De Bruyne B, Bonnier HJ, et al. Long-term follow-up after deferral of percutaneous transluminal coronary angioplasty of intermediate stenosis on the basis of coronary pressure measurement. J Am Coll Cardiol 1998; 31:841–7.

165. Chamuleau SA, Meuwissen M, Koch KT, et al. Usefulness of fractional flow reserve for risk stratification of patients with multivessel coronary artery disease and an intermediate stenosis. Am J Cardiol 2002; 89:377–80.

166. Chamuleau SA, Tio RA, de Cock CC, et al. Prognostic value of coronary blood flow velocity and myocardial perfusion in intermediate coronary narrowings and multivessel disease. J Am Coll Cardiol 2002; 39:852–8.

167. Leon MB, Teirstein PS, Moses JW, et al. Localized intracoronary gamma-radiation therapy to inhibit the recurrence of restenosis after stenting. N Engl J Med 2001; 344:250–6.

168. Teirstein PS, Massullo V, Jani S, et al. Catheter-based radiotherapy to inhibit restenosis after coronary stenting. N Engl J Med 1997; 336:1697–703.

169. Waksman R, White RL, Chan RC, et al. Intracoronary gamma-radiation therapy after angioplasty inhibits recurrence in patients with in-stent restenosis. Circulation 2000; 101:2165–71.

170. Waksman R, Bhargava B, White L, et al. Intracoronary beta-radiation therapy inhibits recurrence of in-stent restenosis. Circulation 2000; 101:1895–8.

171. Waksman R, Raizner AE, Yeung AC, Lansky AJ, Vandertie L. Use of localised intracoronary beta radiation in treatment of in-stent restenosis: the INHIBIT randomised controlled trial. Lancet 2002; 359:551–7.

172. Raizner AE, Oesterle SN, Waksman R, et al. Inhibition of restenosis with beta-emitting radiotherapy: Report of the Proliferation Reduction with Vascular Energy Trial (PREVENT). Circulation 2000; 102:951–8.

173. Sabate M, Costa MA, Kozuma K, et al. Geographic miss: a cause of treatment failure in radio-oncology applied to intracoronary radiation therapy. Circulation 2000; 101:2467–71.

174. Costa MA, Sabat M, van der Giessen WJ, et al. Late coronary occlusion after intracoronary brachytherapy. Circulation 1999; 100:789–92.

175. Teirstein PS, Massullo V, Jani S, et al. Three-year clinical and angiographic follow-up after intracoronary radiation: results of a randomized clinical trial. Circulation 2000; 101:360–5.

176. Kay IP, Wardeh AJ, Kozuma K, et al. Radioactive stents delay but do not prevent in-stent neointimal hyperplasia. Circulation 2001; 103:14–17.

177. Degertekin M, Lemos PA, Lee CH, et al. Intravascular ultrasound evaluation after sirolimus eluting stent implantation for de novo and in-stent restenosis lesions. Eur Heart J 2004; 25:32–8.

178. Colombo A, Hall P, Nakamura S, et al. Intracoronary stenting without anticoagulation accomplished with intravascular ultrasound guidance. Circulation 1995; 91:1676–88.

179. Gorge G, Haude M, Ge J, et al. Intravascular ultrasound after low and high inflation pressure coronary artery stent implantation. J Am Coll Cardiol 1995; 26:725–30.

180. Nakamura S, Colombo A, Gaglione A, et al. Intracoronary ultrasound observations during stent implantation. Circulation 1994; 89:2026–34.

181. Stone GW, St Goar FG, Hodgson JM, et al. Analysis of the relation between stent implantation pressure and expansion. Optimal Stent Implantation (OSTI) Investigators. Am J Cardiol 1999; 83:1397–400, A8.

182. Glagov S, Weisenberg E, Zarins CK, Stankunavicius R, Kolettis GJ. Compensatory enlargement of human atherosclerotic coronary arteries. N Engl J Med 1987; 316:1371–5.

183. Stone GW, Hodgson JM, St Goar FG, et al. Improved procedural results of coronary angioplasty with intravascular ultrasound-guided balloon sizing: the CLOUT Pilot Trial. Clinical Outcomes With Ultrasound Trial (CLOUT) Investigators. Circulation 1997; 95:2044–52.

184. Schroeder S, Baumbach A, Haase KK, et al. Reduction of restenosis by vessel size adapted percutaneous transluminal coronary angioplasty using intravascular ultrasound. Am J Cardiol 1999; 83:875–9.

185. de Jaegere P, Mudra H, Figulla H, et al. Intravascular ultrasound-guided optimized stent deployment. Immediate and 6 months clinical and angiographic results from the Multicenter Ultrasound Stenting in Coronaries Study (MUSIC Study). Eur Heart J 1998; 19:1214–23.

186. Fitzgerald PJ, Oshima A, Hayase M, et al. Final results of the Can Routine Ultrasound Influence Stent Expansion (CRUISE) study. Circulation 2000; 102:523–30.

187. Hoffmann R, Mintz GS, Mehran R, et al. Tissue proliferation within and surrounding Palmaz-Schatz stents is dependent on the aggressiveness of stent implantation technique. Am J Cardiol 1999; 83:1170–4.

188. Bermejo J, Botas J, Garcia E, et al. Mechanisms of residual lumen stenosis after high-pressure stent implantation: a quantitative coronary angiography and intravascular ultrasound study. Circulation 1998; 98:112–18.

189. Serruys PW, Deshpande NV. Is there MUSIC in IVUS guided stenting? Is this MUSIC going to be a MUST? Multicenter Ultrasound Stenting in Coronaries Study. Eur Heart J 1998; 19:1122–4.

190. Johansson B, Allared M, Borgencrantz B, et al. Standardized angiographically guided over-dilatation of stents using high pressure technique optimize results without increasing risks. J Invasive Cardiol 2002; 14:221–6.

191. Reynolds MR, Rinaldi MJ, Pinto DS, Cohen DJ. Current clinical characteristics and economic impact of subacute stent thrombosis. J Invasive Cardiol 2002; 14:364–8.

191a. Regar E, Lemos PA, Saia F, et al. Incidence of thrombotic stent occlusion during the first three months after sirolimus-eluting stent implantation in 500 consecutive patients. Am J Cardiol 2004; 93(10):1271–5.

192. Werner GS, Gastmann O, Ferrari M, et al. Risk factors for acute and subacute stent thrombosis after high-pressure stent implantation: a study by intracoronary ultrasound. Am Heart J 1998; 135:300–9.

193. Watanabe CT, Maynard C, Ritchie JL. Comparison of short-term outcomes following coronary artery stenting in men versus women. Am J Cardiol 2001; 88:848–52.

194. Mehilli J, Kastrati A, Bollwein H, et al. Gender and restenosis after coronary artery stenting. Eur Heart J 2003; 24:1523–30.

195. Moriel M, Feld S, Almagor Y, et al. Results of coronary artery stenting in women versus men: a single center experience. Isr Med Assoc J 2003; 5:398–402.

196. Karrillon GJ, Morice MC, Benveniste E, et al. Intracoronary stent implantation without ultrasound guidance and with replacement of conventional anticoagulation by antiplatelet therapy. 30-day clinical outcome of the French Multicenter Registry. Circulation 1996; 94:1519–27.

197. Nakamura S, Hall P, Gaglione A, et al. High pressure assisted coronary stent implantation accomplished without intravascular ultrasound guidance and subsequent anticoagulation. J Am Coll Cardiol 1997; 29:21–7.

198. Colombo A, Orlic D, Stankovic G, et al. Preliminary observations regarding angiographic pattern of restenosis after rapamycin-eluting stent implantation. Circulation 2003; 107:2178–80.

199. Fujii K, Mintz GS, Kobayashi Y, et al. Contribution of stent underexpansion to recurrence after sirolimus-eluting stent implantation for in-stent restenosis. Circulation 2004; 109:1085–8.

199a. Lemos PA, Saia F, Ligthart JM, et al. Coronary restenosis after sirolimus-eluting stent implantation: morphological description and mechanistic analysis from a consecutive series of cases. Circulation 2003; 108(3):257–60.

200. Sheiban I, Albiero R, Marsico F, et al. Immediate and long-term results of 'T' stenting for bifurcation coronary lesions. Am J Cardiol 2000; 85:1141–4, A9.

201. Bauters C, Hubert E, Prat A, et al. Predictors of restenosis after coronary stent implantation. J Am Coll Cardiol 1998; 31:1291–8.

202. Ho KKL, Senerchia C, Rodriguez O, Chauhan MS, Kuntz RE. Predictors of angiographic restenosis after stenting: pooled analysis of 1197 patient with protocol-mandated angiographic follow-up from 5 randomized stent trials. Circulation 1998; 98:I-362. [abstract].

202a. Lemos PA, Hoye A, Goedhart D, et al. Clinical, angiographic, and procedural predictors of angiographic restenosis after sirolimus-eluting stent implantation in complex patients: an evaluation from the Rapamycin-Eluting Stent Evaluated At Rotterdam Cardiology Hospital (RESEARCH) study. Circulation 2004; 109(11):1366–70.

203. Elezi S, Kastrati A, Neumann FJ, Hadamitzky M, Dirschinger J, Schomig A. Vessel size and long-term outcome after coronary stent placement. Circulation 1998; 98:1875–80.

204. Elezi S, Kastrati A, Pache J, et al. Diabetes mellitus and the clinical and angiographic outcome after coronary stent placement. J Am Coll Cardiol 1998; 32:1866–73.

205. Briguori C, Sarais C, Pagnotta P, et al. In-stent restenosis in small coronary arteries: impact of strut thickness. J Am Coll Cardiol 2002; 40:403–9.

206. Koyama H, Reidy MA. Reinjury of arterial lesions induces intimal smooth muscle cell replication that is not controlled by fibroblast growth factor 2. Circ Res 1997; 80:408–17.

207. Beatt KJ, Luijten HE, de Feyter PJ, van den Brand M, Reiber JH, Serruys PW. Change in diameter of coronary artery segments adjacent to stenosis after percutaneous transluminal coronary angioplasty: failure of percent diameter stenosis measurement to reflect morphologic changes induced by balloon dilation. J Am Coll Cardiol 1988; 12:315–23.

208. Schomig A, Kastrati A, Elezi S, et al. Bimodal distribution of angiographic measures of restenosis six months after coronary stent placement. Circulation 1997; 96:3880–7.

209. O'Neill WW, Serruys P, Knudtson M, et al. Long-term treatment with a platelet glycoprotein-receptor antagonist after percutaneous coronary revascularization. EXCITE Trial Investigators. Evaluation of Oral Xemilofiban in Controlling Thrombotic Events. N Engl J Med 2000; 342:1316–24.

210. Serruys PW, Luijten HE, Beatt KJ, et al. Incidence of restenosis after successful coronary angioplasty: a time-related phenomenon. A quantitative angiographic study in 342 consecutive patients at 1, 2, 3, and 4 months. Circulation 1988; 77:361–71.

211. Roubin GS, King SB, 3rd, Douglas JS, Jr. Restenosis after percutaneous transluminal coronary angioplasty: the Emory University Hospital experience. Am J Cardiol 1987; 60:39B–43B.

212. Kuntz RE, Baim DS. Defining coronary restenosis. Newer clinical and angiographic paradigms. Circulation 1993; 88:1310–23.

213. Reiber JH, van der Zwet PMJ, Koning G, et al. Accuracy and precision of quantitative digital coronary arteriography; observer-, as well as short- and medium-term variabilities. In: Serruys PW, Foley DP, de Feyter PJ, eds. Quantitative coronary angiography in clinical practice. Dordrecht, The Netherlands: Kluwer Academic Publishers, 1994.

214. Huang S, Bjornsti MA, Houghton PJ. Rapamycins: mechanism of action and cellular resistance. Cancer Biol Ther 2003; 2:222–32.

215. Serruys PW, van Hout B, Bonnier H, et al. Randomised comparison of implantation of heparin-coated stents with balloon angioplasty in selected patients with coronary artery disease (Benestent II). Lancet 1998; 352:673–81.

INDEX

acute coronary syndromes (ACS) 24–5,
   35–40
   30-day outcome 37–8
   baseline and procedural characteristics 36,
     37
   interpretation of results 40
   patient population 35–7
   see also acute myocardial infarction
acute gain 21
acute myocardial infarction (MI)
   early safety of SES 35–40
     30-day outcome 37–8, 43
     baseline and procedural characteristics
       36, 37
     interpretation of results 40
     patient population 35–7
   left main coronary artery disease 59, 60,
     61, 65
   long-term outcomes of SES 41–8
     angiographic outcomes 45
     baseline and procedural characteristics
       42, 43
     clinical outcomes 43–4
     interpretation of results 45–8
     patient population 41–2
   post-SES restenosis 45, 152
   predicting adverse events 38
   see also acute coronary syndromes
ADVANCE study 97
adverse cardiac events, major see major
   adverse cardiac events
angina, unstable see acute coronary
   syndromes
angiography, coronary
   in cost-effectiveness analysis 166
   criteria for lesion severity 109
   follow-up, RESEARCH trial 19, 20–1
   see also quantitative coronary angiography
angioplasty, balloon
   after prior CABG 56–7

bifurcation lesions 99
chronic total occlusions 79, 84, 85
post-dilatation of undersized SES see post-
   dilatation of undersized SES
restenosis after 3
right coronary, predicting adverse events
   38
anti-inflammatory effects, sirolimus 7, 8
antiplatelet therapy
   stent thrombosis and 138, 139
   see also aspirin; clopidogrel
ARTS (Arterial Revascularization Therapy
   Study) 69–71
aspirin 18, 138, 157–8
AWESOME trial 56

balloon angioplasty see angioplasty, balloon
Bcl-3 40
BENESTENT trial 132
BENESTENT II trial 132, 166
bifurcation stenting 28, 99–106
   clinical and angiographic findings 100–2
   interpretation of results 102–6
   ostial restenosis after 101–2, 104–5, 144
   patients and techniques 99–100
brachytherapy, vascular (VBT) 3, 113,
   121–2
   SES after failed 114, 120–1, 123
   vs SES implantation 113–14, 115–20,
     122–3
Bx VELOCITY™ stent 5, 6

CABG see coronary artery bypass grafting
cardiac events, major adverse see major
   adverse cardiac events
cardiogenic shock 41
   left main (LM) stenting 60, 61
   predictive value 38, 44
CAVEAT (Coronary Angioplasty Versus
   Excisional Atherectomy trial) I 99

cell cycle, sirolimus actions 7, 8
chronic total occlusions (CTO) 79–85
  clinical and angiographic follow-up 81
  interpretation of results 84–5
  patients and procedures 79–81
clinical studies, early 8–13
clopidogrel 18, 30–1
  acute MI 42, 43, 48
  after repeat SES implantation 157–8
  in-stent thrombosis treatment 116
  long lesion stenting 98
  stent thrombosis and 138
complications
  acute coronary syndromes 37–8
  de novo coronary lesions 30–1
  see also major adverse cardiac events; post-
    SES restenosis; thrombotic stent
    occlusion
coronary artery bypass grafting (CABG),
  prior 53–8
  interpretation of results 54–8
  patients and procedures 53–4
coronary artery lesions, evaluation of severity
  107–8, 109–11
coronary narrowings <50% 107–11
  baseline and procedural characteristics
    108
  clinical outcomes 108–9
  interpretation of results 109–11
  patient population 107–8
cost-effectiveness analysis 165–8
creatinine clearance 49–50
CRUISE study 125
'crush' stenting, bifurcation lesions 99–100,
  105
C-SIRIUS trial 9, 13, 15
  clinical outcomes 12
  length of lesions stented 93
  patients and procedures 10
  post-SES restenosis 141
  quantitative angiography analysis 11
culotte stenting 99, 105
CYPHER™ stents *see* sirolimus-eluting
  stents

death, post-treatment *see* mortality, post-
  treatment
de novo coronary lesions 23–31

baseline and procedural characteristics
  24–5
  clinical outcomes 25–6, 27
  interpretation of results 29–31
  patient population 23–4
  predictors of adverse events 27–8
diabetes mellitus 24–5
  post-SES restenosis 150–1
  recurrent restenosis 160, 161
  risk of adverse events 28, 30
  stent thrombosis 137–8, 139
drug-eluting stents, rationale 4–5

early clinical studies 8–13
edge restenosis 21, 141, 150
  mechanisms 145
  morphology 142, 144
elderly patients 73–5
  baseline and procedural characteristics
    73–4
  clinical outcomes 74, 75
  interpretation of results 75
endothelium-dependent relaxation 40
ERACI II 69
E-SIRIUS trial 9, 13, 15
  clinical outcomes 12
  length of lesions stented 93
  patients and procedures 10
  post-SES restenosis 141
  quantitative angiography analysis 11
EXCITE trial 153

First-In-Man (FIM) study 8, 15, 135
  fast-release formulation 6
  late loss 154
FK506 binding protein (FKBP12) 7–8
fractional flow reserve 109, 111

gender differences, adverse outcomes 28,
  139
GISSOC trial 85
glycoprotein IIb/IIIa inhibitors 18, 25
  acute coronary syndromes/MI 40, 42,
    43, 48
  de novo coronary lesions 30–1
  in-stent thrombosis treatment 116
  post-dilatation of undersized stents
    127

IMPULSE study 97
in-segment restenosis 150
    definition 21
    SES *vs* bare stents 11, 12–13
in-stent restenosis 3–4, 141, 150
    definition 21
    mechanisms 3, 4, 145
    morphology 142–3
    preventive strategies 3–4
    prior CABG surgery 57–8
    SES *vs* bare stents 11, 12–13
    treatment 113–24
        interpretation of results 121–4
        patient population 113–14
        post-SES restenosis 117–20, 123, 150,
            151–2
        SES for failed brachytherapy 120–1,
            122
        SES *vs* brachytherapy 115–20
intra-aortic balloon pumping 41, 60
intravascular ultrasound (IVUS)
    mild coronary stenoses 109, 111
    post-SES restenosis 143, 144
    undersized stents 125, 126, 128, 130

kidney dysfunction, chronic *see* renal
        impairment
kissing stents 99

large coronary vessels 31
late (luminal) loss 21
    SES *vs* bare metal stents 153–6
        angiographic findings 154–5
        interpretation of findings 155–6
        patient population 153
    very small coronary vessels 89, 90–1
left anterior descending (LAD) artery
    multivessel disease involving *see*
        multivessel coronary disease
    post-SES restenosis risk 150, 151
    very long lesions 94
left main (LM) coronary artery disease
        59–65
    clinical outcomes 60–4
    interpretation of results 64–5
    patients and procedures 59–60
left ventricular assist devices 60

long coronary lesion stenting 93–8
    clinical and angiographic findings 94–6
    interpretation of results 96–8
    patients and procedures 93, 94
    predicting adverse events 28, 30, 97,
        150–1
loss index 21

major adverse cardiac events (MACE)
    acute coronary syndromes/MI 37, 38,
        43–4, 45
    bifurcation stenting 101, 106
    chronic total occlusions 81, 84
    coronary narrowings <50% 108–9, 111
    in cost-effectiveness analyses 165, 166
    de novo coronary lesions 25–6, 27, 30
    elderly patients 74, 75
    in-stent thrombosis 116–17, 121, 123
    left main coronary artery disease 61
    multivessel disease 68, 69–71
    post-dilatation of undersized stents
        127–8, 131
    predictors *see* predictors of adverse events
    prior CABG patients 54–5, 56
    randomized trials 12, 13
    RESEARCH registry definitions 18–19
    very long lesions 96–7
    very small coronary vessels 88, 90
    see also complications
mild coronary lesions *see* coronary
        narrowings <50%
mortality, post-treatment
    acute coronary syndromes/MI 37, 43,
        45, 46–7
    de novo coronary lesions 26, 27
    elderly patients 74, 75
    in-stent thrombosis 116, 123
    left main coronary artery disease 61, 65
    renal impairment 50, 51–2
multivessel coronary disease 67–71
    clinical outcomes 68, 69
    elderly patients 73–4
    interpretation of results 69–71
    patient population 67, 68
    predictive value 38
    procedural characteristics 68–9
MUSIC (Multicenter Ultrasound Stenting in
        Coronaries) study 125, 132

myocardial infarction (MI)
  acute *see* acute myocardial infarction
  definition 19
  post SES 26, 27, 44

neointimal proliferation
  in-stent restenosis 3, 4
  mechanism of inhibition by sirolimus 7–8

older patients *see* elderly patients
ostial lesions
  post-SES restenosis 144, 150, 151
  restenosis after bifurcation stenting
    101–2, 104–5, 144
  very small coronary vessels 89, 90, 91

p27Kip1 8
paclitaxel-eluting stents, post-SES restenosis
    157, 159, 160–1
percutaneous coronary intervention (PCI)
  after prior CABG 56–7
  bifurcation lesions 99, 104
  chronic total occlusions 79, 84–5
  see also angioplasty, balloon; sirolimus-
    eluting stents
platelet function 40, 139
poly(butyl methacrylate) (PBMA) 6
poly(ethylene-co-vinylacetate) (PEVA) 6
post-dilatation of undersized SES 28,
    125–32
  angiographic outcomes 128–9
  clinical outcomes 127–8
  interpretation of results 130–2
  left main coronary artery disease 60, 62,
    65
  patients and procedures 126–7
post-SES restenosis 15
  acute MI 45, 152
  bifurcation lesions 101–2, 103, 144
  chronic total occlusions 81, 84, 85
  edge *see* edge restenosis
  in-segment *see* in-segment restenosis
  in-stent *see* in-stent restenosis
  left main disease 62
  morphology and mechanisms 141–5
    interpretation of results 145
    patients and descriptions 141–4
  predictors in complex patients 147–52

clinical and angiographic findings
    149–50
  interpretation of findings 150–2
  patient population 147–9
  treatment 157–61
  clinical and angiographic follow-up
    159–61
  clinical and procedural findings 159
  interpretation of results 161
  patient population 157–8
  very long lesions 94, 95–6, 97
  very small vessels 89–90, 91
  vs restenosis after conventional stents 11,
    12–13, 150, 151, 154
  see also late loss
predictors of adverse events
  acute coronary syndromes/MI 38, 44
  de novo coronary lesions 27–8, 29
  post-SES restenosis 147–52
proliferating cell nuclear antigen 8
psychological questionnaire 19

quantitative coronary angiography (QCA)
    20–1
  acute MI 45, 46
  bifurcation lesions 101–2
  chronic total occlusions 79, 81, 84
  in-stent restenosis 115–16
    SES after failed brachytherapy 121,
      122
    SES *vs* brachytherapy 117–20
  late luminal loss 154–5
  post-dilatation of undersized stents 128–9
  very long lesions 94, 95–6
  very small vessels 89–90
  see also angiography, coronary

radiation therapy, localized vascular *see*
    brachytherapy, vascular
randomized clinical trials 8–13
Rapamycin *see* sirolimus
RAVEL trial 9, 12, 15, 23
  clinical outcomes 12
  cost-effectiveness analysis 165–6
  late loss 154
  length of lesions stented 93
  patients and procedures 10
  post-dilatation of undersized stents 125

post-SES restenosis 141
quantitative angiography analysis 11
simple lesions 109
small coronary vessels 87, 91
vs RESEARCH study 30
regulatory approval, sirolimus-eluting stents
15–16
renal function, evaluation 49–50
renal impairment 49–52
baseline and procedural characteristics
50
interpretation of results 52
one-year outcomes 51–2
patient population 49–50
repeat revascularization
acute MI 44, 45, 47–8
clinically driven 19
in cost-effectiveness analyses 165–6, 167
left main (LM) coronary artery disease
61, 62
multivessel disease 67, 68, 69
post-SES restenosis 157–61
see also coronary artery bypass grafting
(CABG), prior; target lesion
revascularization; target vessel
revascularization
RESEARCH registry 15–21
angiographic follow-up 20–1
complications after SES
late luminal loss 153–6
morphology and mechanisms of
restenosis 141–5
predictors of restenosis 147–52
thrombotic stent occlusion 135–9
treatment of post-SES restenosis
157–61
de novo coronary lesions 23–31
endpoint definitions and clinical follow up
18–19
high-risk patients
acute coronary syndromes 35–40
acute MI 41–8
elderly 73–5
left main (LM) disease 59–65
multivessel disease 67–71
prior CABG 53–8
renal impairment 49–52
patient population 16–17, 18

procedures and post-intervention
medications 18
rationale 15–16
special anatomic groups
bifurcation lesions 99–106
chronic total occlusions 79–85
in-stent restenosis 113–24
mild lesions (narrowings <50%)
107–11
post-dilatation of undersized SES
125–32
very long lesions 93–8
very small coronary vessels 87–91
restenosis
bare metal stents *vs* SES 11, 12–13, 150,
151, 154
in-stent *see* in-stent restenosis
post-angioplasty 3
post-dilatation of undersized SES 128,
129, 131–2
post SES implantation *see* post-SES
restenosis
spot 142
retinoblastoma protein 8
right coronary artery, very long lesions 94,
95–6

saphenous vein bypass grafts 56–8
SES *see* sirolimus-eluting stents
SICCO trial 85
SIRIUS trial 9, 12–13, 15, 23
clinical outcomes 12
cost-effectiveness analysis 166–7
length of lesions stented 93
patients and procedures 10
post-SES restenosis 141, 150–1, 157
quantitative angiography analysis 11
small coronary vessels 87, 91
vs RESEARCH study 30
sirolimus 7–8
carrier vehicle 5, 6
content of stents 7
delivery after stent post-dilatation 125,
130–1
mechanism of action 7–8
release kinetics 6
sirolimus-eluting stents (SES) 5–7
cost-effectiveness 165–8

sirolimus-eluting stents (SES) (*cont.*)
  drug carrier vehicle 5, 6
  drug content 7
  drug release kinetics 6
  metal stent platform 5–6
  rationale 4–5
  regulatory approval 15–16
  sizes 6
small coronary vessel stenting 87–91
  clinical and angiographic follow-up 88,
    89–90
  interpretation of results 90–1
  patients and procedures 87–9
  post-SES restenosis risk 150–1
smooth muscle cells, sirolimus actions 7, 8
SOS (Stent or Surgery) trial 69
spot restenosis 142
stents, coronary
  bare metal *vs* sirolimus-eluting 9–13
  rationale for drug-eluting 4–5
  sirolimus-eluting *see* sirolimus-eluting
    stents
STOP trial 85
survival, post-treatment *see* mortality, post-
  treatment

target lesion revascularization (TLR)
  after treatment of post-SES restenosis 159
  bifurcation lesions 101, 102, 104
  definition 19
  in-stent thrombosis 116–17, 122
  left main (LM) disease 62
  mild lesions (narrowings <50%) 111
  multivessel disease 69
  predictors 27–8, 29
  very small vessels 90
Target of Rapamycin, mammalian (mTOR)
  7–8

target vessel revascularization (TVR)
  definition 19
  de novo coronary lesions 26, 27, 29
  elderly patients 74, 75
  renal impairment 52
  very long lesions 96
thrombotic stent occlusion ((sub)acute stent
    thrombosis; SAT) 135–9
  acute coronary syndromes/MI 37, 38,
    43, 45, 47
  bifurcation lesions 104
  definition 19
  de novo coronary lesions 26, 30–1
  interpretation of results 138–9
  longer stents 98
  mild coronary stenoses 109
  study population and incidence 135–8
TIME (Trial of Invasive *versus* Medical
    therapy in Elderly patients) 75
TOSCA trial 85
T-stenting, bifurcation lesions 99, 103,
    104–5, 144
TULIP study 97

ultrasound, intravascular *see* intravascular
    ultrasound

vascular brachytherapy *see* brachytherapy,
    vascular
vasopressors 41
very long coronary lesion stenting *see* long
    coronary lesion stenting
very small coronary vessel stenting *see* small
    coronary vessel stenting

women, adverse outcomes 28, 139